MW00915114

LOPA Y. GUPTA, M.D.

KILLER FILLER

AND THE

FESTOON PANDEMIC

Saving Face

Illustrations by Jaya Matteis and Kasmira Gupta

Published by 2 Market Media with Dr. Lopa Gupta

ISBN 979 8 396 05903 0

For Dilan,
My precious son
My raison d'etre
My inextinguishable light

TABLE OF CONTENTS

Acknowledgments

Everything I have accomplished in the spirit of decreasing human suffering and improving the lives and livelihoods of my patients here and abroad emanates from my Vedic heritage (*sanskars*) inculcated in me by my loving parents, Yogesh and Mrudula Shah, from the boundless opportunities afforded to an immigrant Indian family by this great country, from its superb educational institutions, and from my extraordinary mentors. In addition, the unconditional love and support I have received from my husband, Mantu, and my children, Sarina, Dilan, and Kasmira have served as my backbone. My gratitude also extends to my devoted staff who have worked tirelessly to provide concierge care for each patient. Lastly, I am indebted to my patients for their trust and confidence in me, inspiring me to challenge traditional routes and pave new roads. Their gracious testimonials have been sprinkled throughout the book as their invaluable feedback has fueled my drive.

Chapter 1
My Back Story

I was born in 1965 in Jhagadia, a small village in Gujarat, India. My father came to the United States in 1969 with a wallet that was empty and a heart that was full of dreams, like so many immigrants before and after him. He came on an academic scholarship to pursue a master's degree in engineering at the University of Pittsburgh. Meanwhile, my mother, brother, sister, and I stayed behind in my uncle's studio apartment in Mumbai from 1969 to 1973. We felt grateful to my uncle for providing us with a roof over our heads. We did not mind sleeping on the kitchen floor in the company of roaches, without any mattresses or pillows–so long as we had my mother's arms and legs. When I was five, we visited my uncle, a village doctor who practiced out of his home. As we approached his house, there stood a long queue of people waiting to see him, their faces riddled with pain and anxiety. The faces of those leaving exuded relief and gratitude. As a young child this visual experience was transformative, and at that very moment I decided that I, too, would like to mitigate the pain and suffering of others one day.

When I immigrated to the U.S. in 1973, I knew full well that without hard work and dedication, my dreams may never come to fruition. Academically, I excelled, but my father had the prescience to broaden my horizons despite his limited resources.

He enrolled me in classical Indian dance, Bharat Natyam, at the age of 11 to infuse Indian culture into me and to develop physical stamina. I also joined my school's field hockey and softball teams. Though at first I despised the drudgery of daily practice, with time I appreciated that mastery of any art form or athletic pursuit demands discipline, perseverance, and passion. Dance tapped into the creative aspect of my personality and sports engrained in me the value and meaning of teamwork. I performed Bharat Natyam at numerous local venues, my stage confidence improving with each dance. The *pièce de résistance* was being selected to perform the leading role of Sita in a dance drama (Ramayana) at Madison Square Garden. Another passion of mine–oddly enough for an athletic teenager–was sewing. I enjoyed creating my own patterns and stitching by hand and machine various dresses and handbags. Little did I realize then how valuable each of these extracurricular pursuits would be in molding me into the creative artist and surgeon I am today.

I graduated in 1983 as class valedictorian with a plethora of scholarships. I credit my school for the excellent education I received but the most unique aspect of Wyomissing High was that it offered a career internship program, a mini apprenticeship to test the waters of a career interest before segueing to college or a technical school. I chose to shadow a local neurosurgeon, Dr. Eric Holm, who illuminated my medical path. I was overwrought with awe and admiration–all at once– as I observed Dr. Holm performing magic in the operating room (OR), from placing a ventriculo-peritoneal (VP) shunt in a child with hydrocephalus to excising a tumor from a child's brain. Vicariously, I felt satisfaction at the instantaneous improvement in the lives of his patients. The thrill of surgery was strikingly familiar to the same "high" I experienced after striking out a player during a softball game or getting a goal in field hockey. To operate on the brain, in the OR, with my own hands, would be a dream come true and the utmost honor for me.

I garnered a spot in Northwestern's competitive Six Year Honors Program in Medical Education (HPME) and was able to save my parents two years' tuition as I would receive my BS/MD degrees in six years. Naturally, I was determined to become a neurosurgeon, until reality struck during my Neurosurgery rotation: up at 6 am for morning rounds, then in the OR from 7 am till 7 pm, followed by evening rounds until 8 pm and in bed by 9 pm– until the next 24 hour cycle. With each passing day, I was becoming increasingly weary for morning rounds and my erect posture in the OR morphed into a slouch by the end of three weeks –and I was just observing! I thought to myself, "How am I going to be a wife and mother one day if I am married to the hospital?" I was completely devastated and felt as if a part of me died. How much more newfound respect and admiration I gained for neurosurgeons–the tremendous personal sacrifices they must make to serve humanity.

As a medical student with goals of saving lives but also raising a family, ideally and ideologically the way my parents raised me, I realized early on that certain professional sacrifices needed to be made. My boyfriend of five years—now my husband—who was also in the HPME suggested I try ophthalmology "as a compromise" for neurosurgery in that the eye is an extension of the brain and that surgery is an integral part of that field as well. I was reluctant at first, but he persisted, and the rest is history. I fell in love with every aspect of ophthalmology—from the OR to the clinic to the research lab. It was certainly no compromise to neurosurgery. Ophthalmology was and remains a rapidly advancing field, with an incredible mix of medicine and microsurgery, numerous subspecialties, as well as cutting-edge research and technology.

During my residency in ophthalmology at Stanford , I had the privilege and honor of training with pioneers and leaders in the field, including Drs. Michael Marmor, Mark Blumenkranz, Peter Egbert, and Kuldev Singh. They taught me how to become an excellent ophthalmic surgeon not only by rote and repetition but by really understanding the core and essence of every diagnosis or surgery, with heavy emphasis on current and established research, thorough knowledge of anatomy, and compassionate patient care. Creating and collaborating on bench research projects with Dr. Marmor throughout my residency taught me the importance of asking questions about unknown concepts and thus, thinking outside the box. This led to several peer-reviewed articles and a book chapter before I finished my residency. I was poised and primed for an academic career in retina, but...

During my final year as Chief Resident, I decided to broaden my horizons and opted to do an elective rotation shadowing Dr. George Paris, an oculoplastic surgeon who had his private office situated in idyllic Palo Alto. I observed various eyelid procedures performed under local anesthesia right in the office while he chatted with the patient and hummed to classical music. These experiences felt more like meditation than anxiety-laden hospital-based surgeries. What a concept! As a resident, I had only experienced operations performed in the OR "theatrical production style," replete with bright lights, props (tubes, catheters, blood pressure cuffs, IV bags), a stage (the OR chair), actors (patient, doctor, anesthesiologist), stagehands (nurses, residents), and an audience (medical students, visiting doctors)— akin to a Broadway show! For me as an impressionable resident, the seed for the allure of office-based surgery was unwittingly planted by Dr. Paris. Off I went to Albany to be trained in oculoplastic and reconstructive surgery by one of the founding fathers of the field, the late Dr. Orkan Stasior.

Dr. Stasior was a force to be reckoned with. Not only was he an incredible anatomist, surgeon, human being, and mentor, but he was a trailblazer. I still remember him grilling me on two very important teaching points: 1) If there is no photograph, it did not happen; and 2) If the surgery does not exist, invent it. As luck would have it, during my fellowship in 1996-97, the U.S. Food and Drug Administration (FDA) approved the Coherent Ultrapulse carbon dioxide (CO_2) laser for blepharoplasty (eyelid surgery), deeming it "safe and effective" [K963339, 510(k)].[1] Dr. Stasior promptly procured a laser and a patient graciously consented to undergo a lower lid blepharoplasty in an unconventional manner: one side with laser and the other with scalpel/scissor. One week later, the scalpel side had deep purple bruising down to the lower face whereas the laser side had a mere yellowish tinge localized to the lower lid. This is because the laser was gentler on the tissues during incision and dissection as it simultaneously cauterized bleeding vessels. This translated to less intraoperative bleeding and decreased postoperative bruising and swelling. Most importantly, it made for safer surgery with less patient downtime. Though my mentor and I were simply dabbling with this exciting new treatment modality, this experience would dictate my career.

I began my practice in 1997, intrigued by laser technology. I performed hundreds of CO_2 laser blepharoplasties during the first few years, and with hard work and "laser" focus, I was able to fine-tune my technique fairly expeditiously. To expand my surgical repertoire, I took intensive and advanced hands-on courses on radio wave surgery, endoscopic brow lifting, liposculpture, and mini face lifting. As my cosmetic eyelid practice burgeoned, I expanded into other avant-garde laser and light treatments. Briefly, LASER is an acronym for Light Amplification by Stimulated Emission of Radiation. In a laser, the lasing medium contains atoms whose orbiting electrons are excited to a higher energy level by a bright light flash. When these excited atoms release their energy, photons are released at a specific wavelength and phase, which excites other atoms. At each end of the lasing medium, a pair of mirrors reflect and amplify the monochromatic (single wavelength) and coherent (waves in the same phase) photons to create a collimated beam of light called a laser. The lasing medium can be solid (e.g., ruby, neodymium:yttrium-aluminum-garnet or Nd:YAG, erbium:YAG or Er:YAG), gas (e.g., CO_2; helium-neon; argon), liquid dye (e.g., rhodamine 6G), or semiconductor (e.g., diode). Light energy, on the other hand, is not monochromatic, coherent, or collimated; multiple wavelengths are emitted by light devices. For each wavelength, there is a target tissue, or chromophore, in the body that absorbs that energy, leading to its partial or complete destruction. Naturally, the goal of rejuvenation is to use the right laser or light device with the appropriate wavelength for controlled and precise destruction of the "unwanted" target tissue. The most common chromophores include water, hemoglobin, and melanin. Thus, I obtained an Er:YAG laser with a wavelength of 2940 nanometers (nm) and chromophore of water to revitalize skin. Water is abundant in our skin cells and heats up upon absorbing the laser energy, causing the cell membrane to rupture. The outer layers of the skin are thus vaporized, prompting the body to lay down new skin that is firmer with more collagen. I added to my armamentarium an Intense Pulse Light (IPL) device. This emits wavelengths in the 500-1200 nm range with hemoglobin and melanin as the target tissues. IPL allowed me to safely treat patients with rosacea who had broken capillaries and redness as well as patients with sunspots or pigmentary disturbances. Lastly, I added a Nd:YAG laser with a wavelength of 1064 nm to target hemoglobin and melanin; this laser enabled me to painlessly and safely perform spider vein and hair removal for all skin types without any risk of burning skin or causing pigmentary changes.

By 2001, my entire practice became cosmetic in nature. To develop myself as an artist and transform my office into a boutique-style studio, I needed an environment that was serene, clean, inspirational, and inviting to patients. As a proud disciple of my mentors at Stanford, Dr. Paris, and Dr. Stasior, I vowed to uphold the highest standards of medical care. I created an office-based surgical suite where performing laser and radio wave surgeries under local anesthesia became not only my studio for creative artwork, but my sanctuary for yoga and meditation as well. Not being beholden to a hospital allowed me to raise three beautiful children and devote myself to being a mother and wife in addition to being a surgeon. I voluntarily withdrew my participation in insurance plans that entail hours of extra work and aggravation. I therefore had plenty of time to properly educate and train my staff on all procedures I offered, enabling them to provide personalized and compassionate care for each patient. Gleaning from my softball and field hockey experiences, I strived for a team approach where every member served a vital role, and every member was *equally* important. There is no "I" in team, and, thus, there existed no hierarchy in my office. For my medical assistants and nurses, training took six months. This included careful observation of each and every step of my procedures followed by surgical assistance supervised by me and another qualified assistant. It was also important for the trainee to memorize by rote the preoperative and postoperative protocols. As my surgeries are performed with local anesthesia and demand optimal concentration and precision, maintaining a "light" atmosphere in the operating suite by playing soothing music and treating the patient in a calm, comforting manner was paramount to relieving stress and anxiety. The front desk staff were also educated on the procedures I offered and instructed to treat each patient with a smile, professionalism, and a heart full of compassion and understanding. Before long, my staff and I were on the same wavelength, and we became a well-oiled machine.

"Dr. Gupta and her staff were fantastic throughout the whole process: consultation, procedure, and follow-up. She has tremendous experience and that eliminated any anxiety. I could not be happier with my results of my upper eyelids. I look refreshed, awake, and recovery was quick."

"If you are looking for a cosmetic procedure, both Dr. Gupta and her staff are masterful. I couldn't be more pleased with their work and the positive atmosphere in the office."

Having established this foothold when I did was key to what was about to happen in the world of cosmetic surgery.

Chapter 2
The Cosmetic Boom

The explosion! Extreme Makeover premiered on national television in 2002, inciting the cosmetic boom. That same year, Botox® was approved by the Food and Drug Administration (FDA) to reduce facial wrinkles, followed by fillers such as Restylane® in 2003, Sculptra® in 2004, and Juvederm® and Radiesse® in 2006. In subsequent years, many more fillers were added to the Restylane® and Juvederm® lineages. Autologous fat injections to the face were also becoming very popular as "natural" fillers. By 2007, according to statistics published by the American Society of Plastic Surgeons (ASPS), 11.7 million cosmetic procedures were performed of which surgical procedures comprised 18% and non-surgical 82%. In the former group, liposuction, breast augmentation, eyelid surgery, facelift, and rhinoplasty were the top five, whereas laser hair removal, chemical peel, Botox®, Restylane®, and microdermabrasion constituted the top five in the latter group. Women underwent 91% of all cosmetic procedures performed. Compared to 1997, there was a 457% increase in total cosmetic procedures; surgical procedures increased by 114% while non-surgical treatments surged by 754%![2]

This cosmetic boom became contagious for doctor and patient alike. Insurance payments were declining, and the captive cosmetic audience was growing by leaps and bounds, leading many physicians and non-physicians to adopt aesthetic procedures into their practices. Before long the cosmetic bandwagon became a clown car teeming with pediatricians, radiologists, anesthesiologists, dentists, dermatologists, gynecologists, family practitioners, plastic surgeons, oculoplastic surgeons (me included), otolaryngologists, nurses, nurse practitioners, and aestheticians to name a few. Every injector aimed to give their patients the fountain of youth by volumizing hollowed under eyes (tear troughs), laugh lines (nasolabial folds), cheeks, lips, and temples. Filler company representatives fueled the fire, claiming that the filler would dissolve in less than a year and that patients should adhere to their annual injection schedules to maintain the look. Fortunately, my cautious, conservative nature and reluctance to follow herd mentality prevented me from over injecting, as eloquently described by this patient:

Janet's story:

"I have been going to Dr. Gupta for years. Under her skilled and compassionate care, I am able to maintain a natural, rested, and more youthful appearance without looking fake or overdone. Dr. Gupta's approach is to never create a different 'you' and she is open and honest about what procedures she does and does not do. She is honest and principled and her aesthetic standards are matched with a great concern for her patients. Together with her talented staff, she has created a wonderful practice that puts patients' safety and needs first. In my years of experience with her, my treatment results have exceeded my expectations, yet have never been overdone. She is consistently honest about what her areas of expertise are. If she feels your personal expectations are at odds with her subtle, natural results, she will gladly recommend you go to a plastic surgeon for deep tissue surgery, which she does not do. Honesty, integrity, skill, and compassion define this talented physician! I trust Dr. Gupta and her staff completely."

Unfortunately, those who succumbed to serial injections elsewhere had so much accumulation of filler that they no longer looked like themselves. To me, they looked so "puffed and stuffed" that they had lost their natural anatomic contouring and their faces demonstrated what I coined "filler dysmorphia." At many a social gathering, dysphemisms such as "chipmunk cheeks," "pillow face," "duck lips," and "cartoon face" resonated. As more and more patients were seeking specialists like me to restore their natural look, I noted that I, as an established oculoplastic surgeon, was being referred an abundance of festoon patients as a consequence of the filler craze.

Chapter 3
The Birth of a Novel Festoon Procedure

By definition, a festoon is "a decorative wreath or garland suspended from two points to form a graceful loop." Situated on the center of the face, just under the eyes, festoons are unsightly cheek mounds and are hardly decorative or graceful! Makeup is ineffective in covering them and they project a chronically tired look to the face, as illustrated in the photograph below.

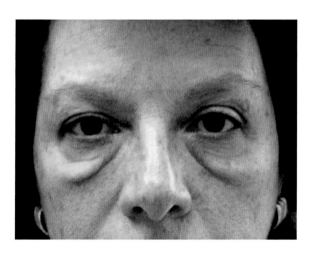

Representative photograph of a patient with hereditary festoons

By 2007, I was seeing a significant number of patients with hereditary festoons exacerbated by filler, as well as de novo festoons caused by filler alone. The culprit in most cases was hyaluronic acid (or HA) fillers such as Juvederm® or Restylane®. In some patients, I was able to reverse the festoon with one or more injections of an enzyme, called hyaluronidase, which dissolved the filler. For festoons resistant to enzymatic degradation, cosmetic surgeons had but two festoon treatment options in their arsenal. One was direct excision of the festoon, entailing a large horizontal scar across the cheek—this was not a viable option for my mostly middle-aged clientele. The other option was aggressive laser resurfacing utilizing either CO_2 or Er:YAG technology.[3] The nuances in the results achieved with these two lasers stem from their differing wavelengths; for CO_2, it is 10,200 nm and for Er:YAG, it is 2,950 nm. Water, which is the chromophore for skin resurfacing, possesses an absorption peak for laser energy at 3,000 nm (see Figure 1), enabling Er:YAG to be much more readily absorbed by the epidermis and papillary (superficial) dermis than CO_2. Conversely, CO_2 can penetrate more deeply into the skin as its path is not as readily impeded by water.

Thus, CO_2 leads to increased thermal damage, collagen stimulation, and coagulation effects. Clinically, however, these enhanced tissue effects translate to more side effects such as prolonged recovery with redness (erythema), severe treatment pain often requiring general anesthesia, and high risk of hypo- or hyperpigmentation. CO_2 laser resurfacing, therefore, was not compatible with my minimal pain and minimal down time philosophy. Understanding laser physics, nonetheless, I did capitalize on the CO_2 laser's superior cutting and coagulation properties, employing it as an incisional tool to perform virtually "bloodless" laser blepharoplasty in office under local anesthesia. For aggressive resurfacing, I preferred Er:YAG technology as it was gentler on the skin with significantly less treatment pain, redness, and pigmentary changes.

FIGURE 1:
ABSORPTION PEAKS FOR WATER

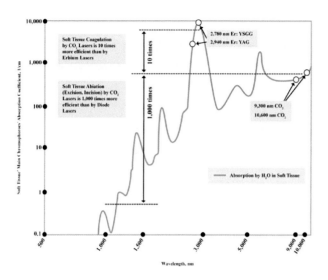

In this graph, the y axis represents the absorption coefficient which is a measure of how much laser energy is lost as it is absorbed by its chromophore (green line—water) per centimeter thickness of soft tissue. The x axis depicts wavelengths in nanometers (nm) along the electromagnetic spectrum. Water has an absorption peak at about 3,000 nm, very close to Er:YAG's wavelength at 2,940 nm, making this laser's absorption coefficient very high (13,000/cm) and ideal for water absorption at the surface with very little deep tissue penetration. CO_2 has a lower absorption coefficient (800/cm), enabling it to maintain enough energy to pass more deeply and exert its superior tissue coagulation effects.

The following patient underwent CO_2 laser upper and lower blepharoplasty in conjunction with aggressive Er:YAG laser resurfacing to treat her upper and lower lid changes and festoons, respectively. As the photographs demonstrate, it was important to address eyelid changes in concert with the festoons for an optimal outcome. While there was an initial "obliteration" of the festoons in the early postoperative period—due to tissue edema after surgery—the festoons began to reappear as the swelling subsided:

PATIENT 1:
ALL PHOTOGRAPHS WITH FLASH

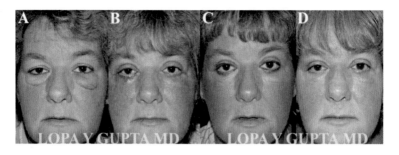

From left to right: (A) The preoperative photograph demonstrates fluid festoons coupled with excess skin and fat in the upper and lower lids. (B) Four weeks after CO$_2$ laser upper and lower blepharoplasty and Er:YAG festoon resurfacing, without makeup. (C) Six weeks postoperative, with makeup. Festoons are "gone." (D) Eight weeks postoperative, without makeup. Postoperative edema is subsiding, but festoons are recrudescing.

PATIENT 1:
PHOTOGRAPHS WITHOUT FLASH

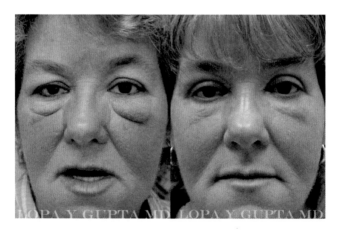

These photographs taken without flash enable better visualization of festoons before surgery (left) and their recurrence as early as eight weeks postoperative after aggressive laser resurfacing (right).

My early experience with Er:YAG resurfacing taught me that this treatment showed partial benefit short-term but I was not convinced of its benefit long-term. If nothing else, it might serve as an adjunctive festoon treatment for larger festoons and a possible treatment for smaller ones.

I felt stuck but had a burning desire to do more to help my festoon patients. Although I had extensive experience in eyelid surgery, I had learned early on that *lower blepharoplasty alone did not correct festoons*, as illustrated by this patient example:

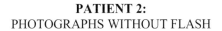

PATIENT 2:
PHOTOGRAPHS WITHOUT FLASH

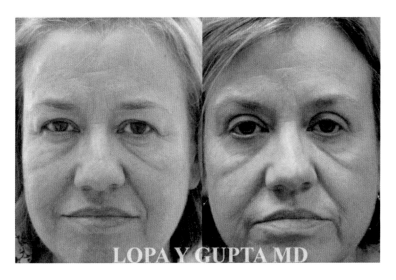

This 61-year-old was bothered by hooded upper lids and baggy lower lids, as seen in the left photograph. The right photograph was taken six weeks after laser upper and lower blepharoplasty with a nice improvement of her eyelid changes, but her "cheek bags" or festoons did not improve after lower blepharoplasty alone—in fact, they looked worse! Since she did not want to go through another procedure, her festoons were managed with camouflage tactics. Her subsequent photographs are demonstrated later in the book, as patient 2.

Putting these pieces of the puzzle together, I knew that I had to address festoons as an entity unto itself, requiring *direct surgical excision and tissue shrinkage*. Moreover, the incision would have to be small and engineered in such a fashion that there would be no visible scar. To achieve this, I would rely on my knowledge of advanced "plastic surgery" suturing techniques and facial surgery principles. Lastly, for optimal precision and safety, I would need to perform the procedure with laser and/or radiosurgery for a technologically advanced but minimally invasive approach, rendering it amenable to an office-based setting under local anesthesia. Adhering to these self-imposed guidelines, I developed a novel festoon technique in 2007—a la Dr. Stasior's axiom, "If it does not exist, invent it." Since festoons occur anatomically in the midface, I felt it apropos to coin my procedure MIDFACE, an acronym for Mini Incision Direct Festoon Access, Cauterization, and Excision.[4] My technique seemed to yield excellent short-term results, and after they were sustained beyond a year, I began posting my festoon work on my website, *www.drlopagupta.com.* Much to my disbelief, within a few years, I became a "festoon specialist" with clients hailing from across the country and around the globe, based on my before and after results. It was remarkable! When asked why they traveled such a distance based on photographic results alone, their response always was that my photographs showed many different angles, short-term and long-term pictures, as well as a natural transformation.

Allison's story:

> *"I was suffering from an under eye condition known as 'festoons'. I had tried different remedies to try and eradicate them, without success. I came across Dr. Lopa Gupta and was so impressed by her experience and knowledge of my condition. I traveled to New York from Australia for my procedure and it was well worth it, as I am absolutely thrilled with the results. I no longer constantly look tired and puffy."*

Patients were also amazed that such a procedure could be performed in the office without going under general anesthesia and that they could fly back home in two to three days. For me, it was validating that patients were appreciating not just my technique and results, but my attention to technology, safe surgery under local anesthesia, and proper photographic representation.

Speaking of photographs, it is noteworthy to mention that truth in photography, especially in my line of work, is essential in obtaining an honest reputation—especially when patients travel large distances for surgery and incur extra expenses. Moreover, it is about practicing good, honest medicine. All too often—be it medical conferences, websites, or laser company representatives with their promotional brochures—I have seen misrepresentation of results with deceptive photography. The before pictures shown are taken with no flash, which makes changes such as scars, eyelid bags, or festoons look worse, and the after photographs are with a flash, which makes results look better. Caveat emptor! It is analogous to comparing an apple with an orange—not fair or accurate. Hypothetically, I can demonstrate a spectacular result—*without any surgery*—by simply placing a no flash photograph as the before and a flash one as the after, even though the pictures are taken seconds apart. As a rule of thumb, the bright flash enters the pupil before it can constrict, strikes the retina, and instantaneously bounces back to the camera which records a distinct, pinpoint pupillary light reflex at the center of the pupil. This reflex is not seen when there is no flash (see following example):

PATIENT 3:
DECEPTIVE PHOTOGRAPHY EXAMPLE

BEFORE | NO FLASH   **AFTER | WITH FLASH**

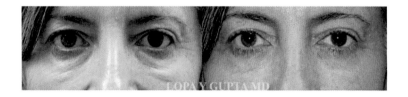

The left photograph is taken without flash and shows prominent festoons. The right photograph, taken with flash, shows "resolution of festoons." Note the pinpoint light reflex in the center of the pupil in the flash photograph. In actuality, the two pictures were taken seconds apart on the same chair, in the same room!

PATIENT 3:
ACCURATE COMPARISON EXAMPLE

BEFORE | NO FLASH   **AFTER | NO FLASH**
ONE YEAR POSTOPERATIVE

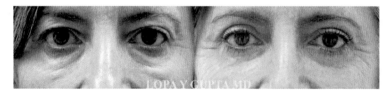

This is an accurate comparison of before and after photographs demonstrating actual results in similar lighting conditions. Both are taken without flash, with the left photograph before surgery and the right one a year after upper/lower blepharoplasty and MIDFACE. Note absence of central pupillary light reflex in both.

Naturally, one would expect improvement after a procedure or laser treatment, but it is difficult to gauge the degree of efficacy if we are not comparing before/after photographs with similar lighting conditions. Such intentional or inadvertent misrepresentation can segue into unrealistic expectations for a patient undergoing a treatment or a physician purchasing a cosmetic laser. This is especially true for festoon patients seeking rejuvenation. The examples below demonstrate representative short-term and long-term results in my patients after eyelid and festoon surgery. The photographs are compared either with flash or without flash, and at different angles:

PATIENT 4:
ALL PHOTOGRAPHS WITH FLASH, FRONTAL VIEW

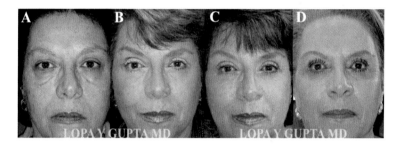

From left to right: (A) A preoperative photograph of a 58-year-old female, demonstrating hereditary festoons, lower eyelid puffiness, and laxity of upper and lower eyelid skin. (B) Nine months after laser upper/lower blepharoplasty and MIDFACE. (C) Four years postoperative with sustained eyelid and festoon improvement. (D) 12 years postoperative with some age-related volume loss along the infraorbital rim and midface regions but a nicely sustained long term result.

PATIENT 4:
ALL PHOTOGRAPHS WITHOUT FLASH, CLOSEUP VIEW

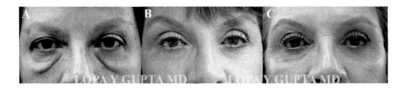

These photographs, without flash, enable better visualization of festoons and eyelid changes. From left to right: (A) is a preoperative, (B) is four years postoperative, and (C) is 12 years postoperative. Note excellent healing of all incision lines and maintenance of the original shape of the eyes.

PATIENT 4
ALL PHOTOGRAPHS WITH FLASH, OBLIQUE VIEW

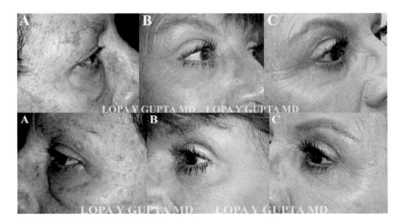

Oblique angle photographs also facilitate visualization of festoon and eyelid changes. From left to right for both rows, (A) is preoperative, (B) is four years postoperative, and (C) is 12 years postoperative.

PATIENT 5:
ALL PHOTOGRAPHS WITH FLASH

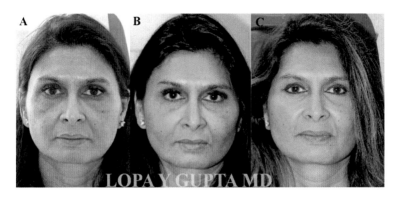

From left to right: (A) Preoperative photograph of a 51-year-old female, demonstrating HA filler-induced festoons causing chronic swelling and pigmentary changes. (B) Six weeks after lower lid blepharoplasty and MIDFACE. (C) One year postoperative with a refreshed look and less discoloration in her lower lids.

PATIENT 5:
PHOTOGRAPHS WITH FLASH, CLOSEUP VIEW

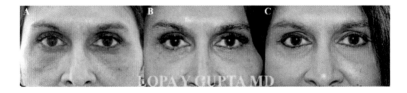

The closeup view allows better visualization of the festoons and lower lid changes. (A) is preoperative, (B) is six weeks after surgery, and (C) is one year postoperative.

PATIENT 5:
PHOTOGRAPHS WITHOUT FLASH WORM'S EYE VIEW

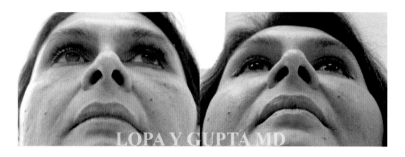

The left photograph demonstrates prominent filler mounds/festoons which are resolved after combined MIDFACE and lower blepharoplasty, as shown in the right photograph.

PATIENT 5:
PHOTOGRAPHS WITHOUT FLASH, OBLIQUE VIEW

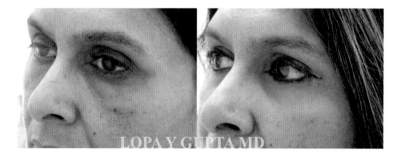

This oblique angle also nicely demonstrates HA filler festoons with associated lower eyelid changes in the left photograph, which are improved after surgery, as shown in the right photograph. Note absence of scarring or change in the shape of her eyes.

PATIENT 5:
INTRAOPERATIVE PHOTOGRAPHS

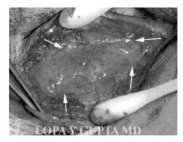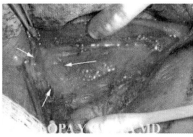

These photographs were taken during a combined MIDFACE and lower lid blepharoplasty procedure. The left one demonstrates the gelatinous, encapsulated HA filler enveloping the medial and central orbital fat pads (arrows). The right photograph shows HA filler (arrows) behind the septum, smothering the lateral orbital fat pad in this patient. This trapped filler, resistant to enzyme, was causing festoons, chronic swelling issues, and pigmentary eyelid changes in this patient. These photos also demonstrate the importance of performing the lower lid procedure to obtain full access and removal of the filler-fat pad complexes for optimal resolution of festoons.

Chapter 4
The Festoon Conundrum

Believe it or not, we are amidst a festoon pandemic as the incidence of festoons has rapidly risen and continues to escalate due to the surge in aesthetic treatments, especially near the eyes. Unfortunately, thousands of afflicted patients are suffering silently worldwide because the diagnosis of festoons is falling through the cracks for a variety of reasons. First, there is confusion about the exact name as numerous aliases exist, including malar mounds, malar edema, malar bags, cheek bags, and festoons! Second, many patients are not aware that their condition even bears a name and consequently, have no starting point with which to begin their search on the internet. Third, many doctors and paramedical injectors are not aware of the existence of this entity and dismiss it when a patient presents with this condition. Fourth, doctors who are familiar with this condition likely do not know how to treat festoons and incorrectly advise patients that there is no remedy for this chronic condition. Fifth, doctors who are aware of treatment possibilities will shy away from management because established festoon repair techniques are extremely difficult to perform, are aggressive in nature, and tend to carry high recurrence and complication rates. Sixth, some injectors "treat" festoons by camouflaging them with hyaluronic acid (HA) fillers or autologous fat grafts, which, in fact, are the absolute worst recipe for a festoon patient. HA fillers and fat may soften the appearance of festoons short-term but can be disastrous long-term. Finally, there are specialists who unwittingly manage festoons by lower lid blepharoplasty alone which only serves to exacerbate them. Consequently, festoons are under-diagnosed, mis-diagnosed, mismanaged, and often left untreated. This has led to a vicious cycle with festoon prevalence increasing hand in hand with significant patient suffering on an emotional, psychological, social, financial, and physical level over the past two decades.

Control of the festoon pandemic begins with heightened awareness of this enigmatic entity as well as all treatment options, on the part of the doctor and patient. Perhaps a single word such as "festoon" be adopted to collectively represent the different aliases so that awareness and further research becomes a simpler process for the patient, doctor, and researcher. Lastly, it is imperative for injectors to prevent festoons or their exacerbation by recognizing that HA fillers and fat grafts (described in more detail later in this book) around the lid/cheek complex persist in the patient permanently and can cause festoons years after injection.

The following testimonials and photographs transform my words to representative, real-life patient experiences.

Diane's Story:

> *"I have spent years searching for the right physician to assist me with correction of improper filler placement and droopy under eyes. I had a blepharoplasty by another physician a few years earlier that did not resolve the issue [festoons]. Dr. Gupta listened, took a thorough history, and identified what the problem was. She solved it! All old filler was removed, eye bags removed, and skin tightened. She and her staff were so caring and gentle. I highly recommend Dr. Gupta. I would give her 10 stars."*

Leigh Ann's Story:

"About four years ago, at age 41, I began to develop the most difficult kind of festoons—some loose skin, but also severe malar/cheek edema. It was in part genetic—several family members have aged this way. However it was aggravated by tear trough fillers I had done five years ago, and in addition to the festoons, I had an odd lump under my left eye which was almost certainly due to the filler. Zero fat pad prolapse—that wasn't my problem. I did CO2 laser resurfacing for the excess skin. It definitely helped, but the malar edema persisted, and I looked 55 years old, not 44. I consulted with seven plastic surgeons in my hometown. Most recommended a) transconjunctival lower bleph and/or b) more filler. A couple of them (very much to their credit) told me they couldn't help me at all, malar edema being notoriously difficult to treat. A shocking couple of them misidentified my problem as fat pad prolapse, even though bags were mostly down on my cheeks. I then flew to NY to see Dr. Gupta. At my consultation with Dr. Gupta, she listened very closely to my explanations, looked very closely at pictures I brought to the consultation, thoroughly/directly examined my eyes from multiple angles, and asked a ton of questions (eg, "what happens to them when you get on a plane?"). I was clear with her that I had no tolerance for over-correction (I don't need to look 15 years younger...I just wanted to look great for 44, but most importantly still look like myself). In turn, she was very clear with me on possible outcomes: this is not a layup, which is why many surgeons won't do it at all. She set very realistic expectations, and I chose her with confidence. Dr. Gupta did not disappoint. I had open lower bleph and direct festoon excision, a painless, excellent experience in the office. And most importantly, I look great two months later. Like myself, but better. Scars aren't invisible just yet, but still even with open procedures, I looked great by 30 days, and even better at 60. Her staff is also fantastic. They explained everything, answered my incessant questions patiently and knowledgeably, made the whole process seamless, and kept my husband comfortable and informed as he waited for me. Highly recommend.

PATIENT 6:
PHOTOGRAPHS WITH FLASH, OBLIQUE VIEW

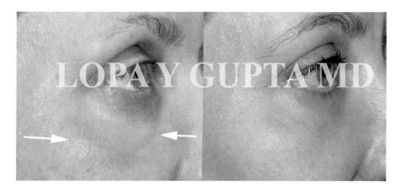

The left photograph delineates the hereditary festoon exacerbated by HA fillers (area between arrows). The right photo demonstrates significant improvement of the festoon just two months after lower blepharoplasty and MIDFACE.

PATIENT 6:
PHOTOGRAPHS WITHOUT FLASH, WORM'S EYE VIEW

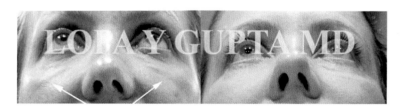

This view with no flash photography clearly demonstrates bilateral festoons (arrows) that are significantly improved 2 months after surgery. The result will evolve as healing progresses over a year.

Chapter 5
Understanding the Festoon Sufferer

For the festoon sufferer, it is depressing to see a tired face in the mirror *every* morning of *every* day. Some mornings, the face is unrecognizable from excessive swelling after an evening of alcohol or salty food. In addition, allergy attacks, an upper respiratory infection, pet handling, air travel, exercise, or sun exposure may exacerbate festoon swelling issues. Comments such as, "you should get more sleep and rest," from friends, family, and co-workers can be draining and demoralizing, especially after a good night's sleep! To camouflage and cope, patients often hide behind rimmed glasses. Thus, festoons detract significantly from the quality of life *on a daily basis.*

Festoons pose more than just a cosmetic problem. They impose a significant financial burden as thousands of dollars are fruitlessly expended on lotions, potions, makeup, consultations, and incorrect treatments. Moreover, patients' mental health may be adversely affected, prompting some to seek psychiatrists, therapists, and medications for sequelae such as depression, anxiety, panic attacks, or substance abuse—further augmenting the financial toll. Productivity at home and at work may be greatly reduced leading to more economic woes.

Many sufferers feel stuck, especially after numerous specialists with whom they have consulted turn them away. All too often, patients are incorrectly advised, "This is a chronic condition and there is no treatment for it—it is something you will just have to live with." This leads to loss of hope and self-esteem. For some, this may segue into depression and social isolation, abandoning their friends, family, and employment. Relationships may be adversely affected or broken. This vicious, negative cycle may go on for years. It is of paramount importance that the festoon specialist be cognizant of these multiple layers and approach the sufferer with sensitivity, compassion, and patience. Most importantly, the *surgeon must serve as the patient's beacon of hope and guiding light* through this complex labyrinth.

Beth's story:

"Over the last several years, I developed large dark bags under my eyes. I began to look tired even though I had plenty of energy. Many of my clients remarked that I looked very exhausted. I even heard comments like, 'It looks like you need a good night's sleep.' I knew they were reacting to my eyes. I tried topical treatments, concealers, coverups, and creams which either didn't help or only made it look worse.

I consulted with Dr. Lopa Gupta, and she recommended two procedures that would address my problem — a lower lid blepharoplasty and direct festoon repair. Dr. Gupta showed me before and after pictures of similar cases and I was sold. Just two weeks after the surgery, I already look so much better. The surgery was a success. My eyes are continuing to improve over time and I couldn't be happier. I highly recommend Dr. Gupta. She is an expert's expert in her field. She made me feel comfortable and reassured, and her staff is excellent. She is now on my short list of trusted medical practitioners."

Currently, there exist only a handful of surgeons worldwide who are adept at surgically treating festoons, albeit through known aggressive techniques. At the time of this writing, MIDFACE is the only minimally invasive festoon surgery of its kind, having withstood the test of time with respect to its efficacy and longevity over the past 15 years. As a disclaimer, the vast majority of my surgical patients include healthy men and women in their 40's, 50's, and 60's. As such, MIDFACE in concert with a lower blepharoplasty when indicated, serve as successful stand-alone procedures for festoons of all sizes in my clientele, as evidenced by these illustrative patient examples:

PATIENT 7:
ALL PHOTOGRAPHS WITH FLASH, FRONTAL VIEW

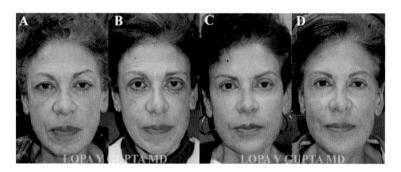

From left to right: (A) Preoperative photograph of a 56-year-old female, depicting fluid festoons from nasal and sinus disease despite medical management. Also evident are upper and lower lid changes. (B) Two weeks after MIDFACE and upper/lower blepharoplasty with presence of mild swelling and bruising. (C) One year postoperative with a refreshed look which is maintained in (D) three years later.

PATIENT 7:
ALL PHOTOGRAPHS WITHOUT FLASH, FRONTAL VIEW

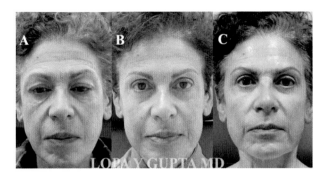

Photography without flash makes it easier to discern festoon and eyelid changes before surgery and their improvements after surgery. (A) is preoperative, (B) is one year after surgery, and (C) is three years postoperative. She also underwent neuromodulator injections to smooth out forehead wrinkles and Radiesse® injections (supraperiosteal) to enhance cheek and midface volume.

PATIENT 7:
ALL PHOTOGRAPHS WITHOUT FLASH, OBLIQUE VIEW

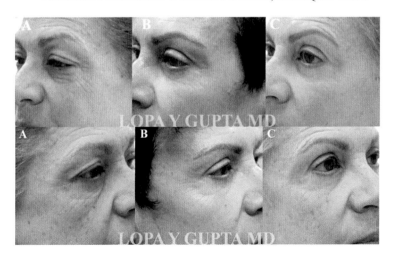

From left to right for both rows: (A) is preoperative, (B) is one year postoperative, and (C) is three years postoperative.

39

PATIENT 8:
ALL PHOTOGRAPHS WITH FLASH

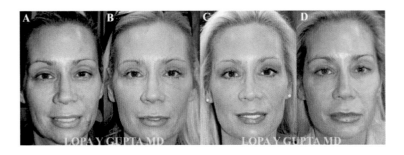

(A) Preoperative photograph of a 44-year-old female with HA filler festoons refractory to enzyme injections as well as age-related upper and lower eyelid changes. (B) Seven weeks postoperative. (C) Seven months postoperative. (D) Five years postoperative. Flash photography makes it more difficult to visualize festoons before and after surgery, reinforcing the need for no flash and angle photography for optimal assessment.

PATIENT 8:
PHOTOGRAPHS WITHOUT FLASH

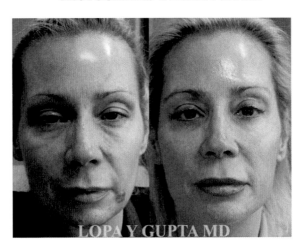

Eyelid changes and festoons are more readily seen in no flash photography. The left photograph is preoperative and the right one is five years postoperative.

PATIENT 8:
ALL PHOTOGRAPHS WITH FLASH, OBLIQUE VIEW

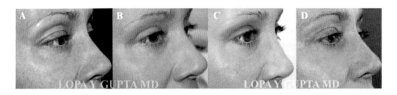

From left to right: (A) Preoperative, showing the festoon along with upper and lower lid changes. (B) Seven weeks postoperative. (C) Seven months postoperative. (D) Five years postoperative. The other side demonstrated similar results.

For patients who are older or who have comorbidities such as diseases of the heart, kidneys, liver, or thyroid gland, MIDFACE may serve as an adjunctive procedure to more aggressive, standard festoon repair techniques.

The testimonials below from my gracious patients bring to light many of the points discussed above.

Sara's Story:

"I had eye surgery with Dr. Gupta and already I am thrilled. Removal of festoons and a lower bleph (had original bleph done 20 years ago with another surgeon). It has only been eight days since surgery and the improvement is already astonishing. Dr. Gupta and her staff (Ann, Amelia, etc.) are simply awesome. You don't need to be a celeb or have tons of money to be treated with respect and the utmost care. I had gone for several consults with other surgeons on how to improve and resolve my eye issues and not one of them except Dr. Gupta made any sense on their recommendations. I would highly recommend a consult with this team if you are having issues with your eyes."

Ken and Denise's Story:

"Over a period of three years, my wife and I had spoken to a couple of surgeons that do cosmetic eye surgery. Her concern was the 'bags' [festoons] under her eyes, and my issue was my heavy upper lids. The inability to find a doctor that we felt comfortable with delayed our procedures. During a business flight, my wife read an article about Dr. Gupta that was very favorable. When we reached out, she answered all of our questions and gave us concise information about our procedures of interest. She was warm, kind, knowledgeable, and seemed to have the education and experience that we were looking for. Besides all of that, she seemed to approach her work with the passion and eye of an artist. We feel very positive about 'our look,' our treatments, and the exceptional care that we received from Dr. Gupta and her amazing staff."

Elizabeth's Story:

"Based on the circumstances of my life these last several years, Dr. Gupta has allowed me to be a part of an experience I had not been able to even imagine I would have again, a feeling of being a 'normal' woman with 'normal' concerns about her looks. Having the good fortune, by happenstance, to meet her, has allowed me to feel better about my life as a whole again. Her compassion, coupled with unsurpassed skill and competence, has allowed me to experience hope about what each day can bring! Thank you, Dr. Gupta! I pray that the world has more medical professionals like yourself and I am grateful to say you are the best!"

After the honor and privilege of being Elizabeth's doctor for 15 years, she succumbed to a chronic disease and left us in 2022. For us, she will always be with us. May her soul rest in peace.

Chapter 6
Festoon Anatomy and Pathophysiology

Festoon Anatomy:

Furnas first described festoons from a weakened orbicularis muscle in 1978.[5] Subsequent to that paper, Kikkawa (1996),[6] Pessa (1997),[7] Mendelson (2002),[8] and Muzaffar (2002)[9] published sentinel papers eloquently detailing the surgical anatomy of the lower eyelids and midface, described below. These studies laid the foundation for a deeper understanding of festoon formation.

"Festoon" is a catch-all term for any excessive sagging, swelling, or fullness present in the lid-cheek junction (LCJ), the area just under the bone of the lower eyelid (infraorbital rim or IOR) and along the top part of the cheek (the malar area). If one palpates this bone beginning at the nose and follows it to the outer part of the eyelid, one will note that it is shaped like a crescent. The ligament that lines this bone along the IOR is called the orbicularis retaining ligament (ORL) or orbitomalar ligament (OML), which is also arcuate or crescent-shaped. The ORL is not very strong, allowing loose, excess lower eyelid skin and/or muscle to cascade down into the upper cheek area. The ORL is also permeable, allowing pressure-assisted leakage of fluids into the malar region. Gravitational descent of tissue and fluid down the face is prevented by a natural wall, called the zygomatic cutaneous ligament (ZCL). This ligament is strong and not permeable, forming a robust barrier (see diagram below). Thus, sagging skin and muscle will drape over the LCJ, like a "decorative" festoon suspended from the ZCL. If there is a fluid component, called edema, the ZCL will act like a dam, creating a reservoir of fluid.

Festoon formation notwithstanding, the ZCL does, however, serve an important role in the face. It is etiologically there to prevent upward spread of infections from the mouth to the eyelids and eyes, through which the pathogen(s) would have easy access to the brain.

The area contained within the boundaries of the ORL and the ZCL is called the prezygomatic space, or the PZS. It is within this space the festoon formation occurs. The different layers of the PZS (from superficial to deep) include skin, subcutaneous fat (also called the malar fat pad), orbicularis muscle, superior part of the suborbicularis oculi fat (SOOF), malar septum, supraperiosteal fat (this lies right over the maxillary sinus), periosteum, and potential space *throughout* (see Figure 2). This potential space acts like a sponge and creates a "sink" for fluid accumulation and festoon formation.

FIGURE 2:
CROSS SECTION OF THE PREZYGOMATIC SPACE

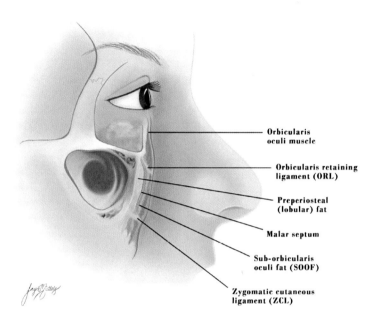

Orbicularis
oculi muscle

Orbicularis retaining
ligament (ORL)

Preperiosteal
(lobular) fat

Malar septum

Sub-orbicularis
oculi fat (SOOF)

Zygomatic cutaneous
ligament (ZCL)

Age-related or senescent festoons typically occur from laxity due to loss of elasticity and thinning of collagen. This, coupled with gravitational descent, can result in cascading or overhanging of any or all of the anatomic structures above the ZCL, including skin, muscle, the ORL, and fat. With edema, the PZS, with its potential space throughout, transforms into a sponge or sink, allowing the fluid to fill the empty reservoirs or holes. Depending on the amount of edema, the sponge can become saturated, or even super-saturated wherein all layers of the PZS become fluid-laden! Thus, the shape of the festoon may range from a thin fluid line to a ridge to a crescent-shaped mound to complete swelling from the lower eyelid margin to the ZCL.

Festoon Pathogenesis:

The next logical question would be: What causes fluid to accumulate in the PZS? If we use the analogy of a sink (see Figure 3), then the fluid level in the sink will rise by turning on the faucet, blocking the drain, or both.

FIGURE 3
THE FESTOON SINK

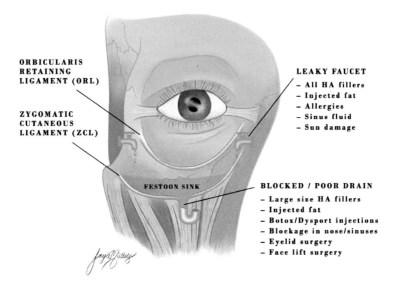

Sources of increased fluid influx (leaky faucet) include:

1) **Inflammation**, both acute and chronic, can cause blood vessels in the eyelid and cheek area to dilate and become leaky (permeable). This results in an outpouring or extravasation of various inflammatory mediators that attract more immune cells leading to tissue swelling and fluid deposition. Inflammatory triggers include:
   • Allergies (environmental, food, pets, medications)
   • Thyroid Eye Disease

- Hyaluronic Acid (HA) Filler
- Autologous Fat Grafts
- Poly-L-Lactic Acid (Sculptra®)
- Silicone
- Sunlight

2) **Hyaluronic acid (HA) fillers** such as Restylane®, Juvederm®, or Voluma® are very hydrophilic (water-loving) and have the ability to significantly contribute to the festoon sink. In fact, each molecule of HA can attract up to 1,000 molecules of water!

3) **Leakage from newly formed blood vessels** (neovascularization) is another source of fluid influx into the PZS. Injected autologous fat is a "live" graft which means that for it to survive and not get resorbed or metabolized by the body, it must establish its own blood supply that courses through it. These new vessels, or neovascularization, do not have strong vessel walls and tend to be leaky (personal intraoperative observation). This seepage thus adds fluid to the sink, engendering festoons in many a fat graft recipient.

4) **Fluid potentiators or "enablers"** such as salt, alcohol, and low atmospheric pressure enhance the osmotic gradient, leading to more fluid deposition. Sufferers often experience significant enlargement of their festoons when they are on a plane or skiing, or after an evening of salty food or alcohol.

5) **Excess sinus fluid** can extravasate into the lower lid/cheek area from a condition called chronic rhinosinusitis (CRS), which can engender or exacerbate festoons. The nasal or sinus inflammation in CRS may be caused by allergies, asthma, or nasal polyps and persists for more than 3 months.

The following is a testimonial from a patient who experienced consequences after silicone injections near the eyes and cheeks. His before/after photographs are also included.

Frank's Story:

"Dr. Lopa Gupta is a superb surgeon. About seven years ago, in 2012, Dr. Gupta removed my eye bags using a laser. It went beautifully. Zero pain, zero complications. Then, in 2017, after I foolishly allowed a famous NYC dermatologist to inject silicone microdroplets in my face, it was Dr. Gupta who removed them after those "droplets" turned into hard red bumps. And lastly, just a few weeks ago, in 2019, I had Dr. Gupta resurface my under eye areas. It went great. After four days, with no down time and sunglasses on, my eye area looks like it belongs to someone 30/35 (and I'm 76). Save yourself any regrets; entrust your eyes and face to Dr. Lopa Gupta."

PATIENT 9:
PHOTOGRAPHS WITH FLASH, CLOSEUP VIEW

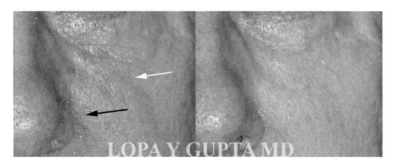

The photograph on the left depicts silicone nodules inciting an inflammatory reaction with a resultant nasal festoon (white arrow) and a hypervascular response extending down near the ala of the nose (black arrow). The photograph on the right is taken after surgical removal of the nodules, MIDFACE, and laser resurfacing.

The next testimonial and set of photographs is from a patient who suffered from HA filler festoons.

Hannah's Story:

"I just want to say Dr. Gupta is the nicest and kindest doctor I have ever met in my life! I visited her yesterday for lower bleph and festoon repair all the way from the UK. I was so nervous, but the whole thing was painless and actually I really enjoyed going there to get it done! The girls there are so lovely and they talked to me throughout the whole procedure. After the procedure they then applied a tape to prevent swelling and gave me a bag full of aftercare products. The clinic itself is also immaculate and luxurious and they will provide you with a VIP service. I have been suffering with this problem for two years following filler injection somewhere else and I had been told by multiple doctors that there was no cure. I'm now just enjoying my time in New York with minimal swelling and no pain! Will be back all the time now to see Dr. Gupta, as she offers a wide range of amazing treatments! I would definitely say you can 1000000% put your trust in this lovely lady as she has an eye for perfection and detail!"

PATIENT 10:
PHOTOGRAPHS WITH FLASH, OBLIQUE VIEW

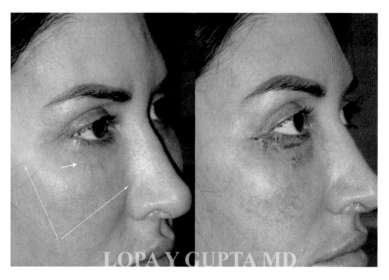

The left photograph demonstrates an expansive HA filler festoon, spanning from the nose to the lateral cheek (long white arrows). Also note the hypervascularity incited by the HA filler that is visible even through the thin lower lid skin (small arrow). The right photograph was taken five days after lateral lower blepharoplasty and MIDFACE. Though it is still early recovery with bruising and swelling, there is already improved contouring. Correspondence with this patient one year later confirmed complete resolution of the festoon with "invisible" lines.

PATIENT 10:
PHOTOGRAPHS WITH FLASH, WORM'S EYE VIEW

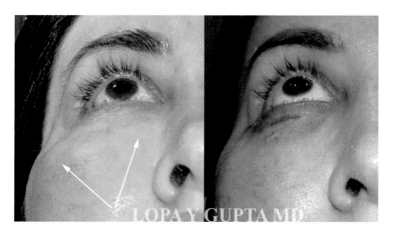

The left photograph demonstrates a broad HA filler festoon with improvement shown in the right photograph 5 days after the procedures. She flew back to the UK with minimal swelling and bruising.

Sources of decreased fluid efflux (blocked or impaired drain):

1) **Weakened orbicularis muscle pump** from aging, neuropathy, or neuromodulator injections[10](Botox®, Dysport®, Xeomin®). The orbicularis muscle encircles the upper and lower eyelid like an onion and when it contracts, it helps squeeze out and drain extra tissue fluid from the eyelids/PZS into the veins and lymphatics. When orbicularis muscle function is compromised, it can add fluid to the festoon sink.

2) **Blocked sinuses or nasolacrimal duct.** The nasolacrimal duct (tear duct) as well as four sinuses that surround the eyes all drain into the nose. Thus, any obstruction in the nose, sinuses, or tear ducts may lead to a backup of fluid into the eyelids and PZS.

3) **Physical impediment of orbital lymphatics** by large quantities of fillers or injected fat placed in the tear trough or lid-cheek junction.

4) **Inadvertent damage to lymphatics** by aggressive facelift, midface lift, or eyelid surgery. Lymphatic drainage of the inner part of the eyelid as well as the sinuses (ethmoid, frontal, maxillary) is mediated by the submandibular lymph nodes whereas the drainage of the outer half of the eyelids, conjunctiva (clear membrane inside eye), and cheek is mediated by the preauricular lymph nodes (Figure 4).

FIGURE 4:
LYMPHATIC DRAINAGE OF THE FACE

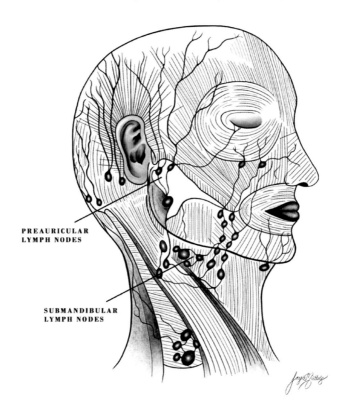

PREAURICULAR
LYMPH NODES

SUBMANDIBULAR
LYMPH NODES

Thus, festoon formation tends to be multifactorial in nature. Not only do certain factors cause both increased influx *and* decreased outflow (a "double whammy") but they often coexist with other triggers, making it an arduous task for the specialist to diagnose and manage festoons effectively. It is no wonder that most doctors do not wish to navigate such a complex labyrinth!

Chapter 7
Proper Festoon Evaluation and Surgical Planning

My typical festoon patient has been suffering for years and is emotionally broken and desperate. I am likely their fifth or sixth consultation after a string of disappointing visits with local plastic surgeons, dermatologists, and other specialists. It is of vital importance for me to gain my patient's trust and I can only do so if I project confidence in my work, show compassion for their suffering, and infuse some semblance of hope right from the outset. Only then can the patient and I really *connect*. During the first few minutes, I assess the patient's face, festoons, and mindset. At the risk of sounding overconfident, I calmly state to the patient that their years of suffering may likely end with me. This immediately puts them at ease, and many begin to cry upon hearing these words. I then listen to each patient's story with patience and alacrity, making direct eye contact throughout.

My consultation continues with a thorough review of any relevant medical conditions (such as sinus or nasal disease, thyroid disease, seasonal allergies); social history (smoking, sun exposure, alcohol use); medications (including antidepressants); family history of festoons; prior surgical history (such as facelift, blepharoplasty, rhinoplasty); history of sleeping with pets; history of any previous facial injectables (such as neurotoxins, fillers, fat grafts). Patients often forget about injectables done years prior or feel that they have "worn off by now" which is NOT the case—an injectable (especially an HA filler) performed under the eye can, in significant proportions, persist for a lifetime, causing chronic festoons if not treated. Moreover, it is important to know if there is any diurnal fluctuation in the size of the festoons. Are they larger in the evening or when first awakening in the morning? Lastly, what triggers tend to exacerbate the festoons? Salt? Alcohol? Flying on a plane? Skiing? Allergies? Sinuses? An upper respiratory infection? The festoon specialist, like a detective, needs to gather all pieces of the puzzle before putting them all together and making sense out of every patient's presentation.

For a proper physical examination of festoons, it is important to have good lighting, magnification, and a face cleaned of makeup. Before zeroing in on the festoons, I first evaluate the presence of previous injections. Telltale signs may include hard nodules from Sculptra, lumps from injected fat grafts, "poofy" cheeks from Voluma® or Juvederm®, or a Tyndall effect from HA fillers (a blue-green discoloration caused by scatter of reflected light from HA particles just under the thin eyelid skin). Absence of smile lines around the eyes (crow's feet) may indicate a weakened orbicularis muscle pump from strong doses of neuromodulators (Botox®, Dysport®, Xeomin®). In addition, scars from prior eyelid or facial surgery may be clues to possible lymphatic damage. Sun damaged skin may also be a contributing factor to festoon formation. Since tear ducts and sinuses drain into the nose, a watery eye, a deviated nasal septum, nasal congestion, or sinus tenderness could impute a blockage in these pathways with resultant backup of fluid into the thin eyelid skin and pooling in the malar areas.

Examination of the festoons should include visualization from various angles (i.e., frontal, oblique, worm's eye view) to assess size and projection, as well as palpation (after washing my hands—I like to feel without gloves) to assess if there is a fluid, solid, or mixed component to the festoons. I have also been using high frequency ultrasound technology to determine the presence of filler if my manual and visual examination are inconclusive.

Lastly, the lower eyelids and festoons should be assessed as a single aesthetic unit, as excess eyelid skin, muscle, or orbital fat (eyelid bags) must be addressed in conjunction with skin, muscle, or fat changes in the gravitationally dependent malar region—treating one may make the other look worse. Taking it a step further, it is important to assess the status of the upper eyelids/brows as well. After my examination, I review a basic facial anatomy diagram and then hand the patient a mirror demonstrating all significant findings so that the patient can see what I see.

Lastly, I formulate a tailored treatment plan, based on the history, review of systems, medications, and physical examination. This often entails a multi-disciplinary approach that recruits the expert help of 1) an allergist or internist to evaluate for and treat seasonal, food, or pet allergies; 2) an Ear Nose Throat (ENT) Surgeon to diagnose and treat any underlying sinus or nasal disease; 3) an endocrinologist to manage thyroid disease. Thus, it behooves the patient to try 3-6 months of any treatment recommended by such specialists—be it medications (i.e., antihistamines, decongestants, corticosteroids, nasal sprays, thyroid meds) or home remedies (i.e., cold compresses, nasal irrigation with netty pots, humidifiers). It is also beneficial for the patient to modify certain habits such as washing their hands after pet-handling, reducing salt and alcohol intake, and optimizing sun protection (sunscreen, hats, glasses). In those who have festoons induced by HA filler under the eyes or cheeks, it is worthwhile to try a reversing enzyme, hyaluronidase, to dissolve the filler first.

Any procedure recommended by an ENT specialist (i.e., balloon sinuplasty, polyp removal) must be done *before* any festoon repair is considered, as festoons may disappear or improve after such intervention. If festoons become more manageable and concealable with makeup, then festoon surgery may be deferred. Here is one patient's experience:

Hope's Story:

> *"I have been a patient of Dr. Gupta for a little over two years now and all I can say is I'm so glad I found her. She helped me gain my confidence back. When I first came to her, I had severe sinus issues that caused me to develop festoons. The swelling under my eyes was very noticeable and I was so uncomfortable with the way I looked. From the moment I met Dr. Gupta, she reassured me that she would help me find a way through this and that there was hope for me to achieve long-lasting, natural results. With her recommendation of first sinus surgery to help with my problem from within, and throughout the healing process, she didn't once pressure me for any quick fixes or surgeries I didn't need to solve my problems with short-term results. After my recovery from sinus surgery, I had several appointments with Dr. Gupta to monitor my progress, along with sessions of laser resurfacing and micro-needling. Through all this, now I'm happy to say I have seen dramatic improvement in my festoon area. Though it's still a work in progress like anything, the swelling under my eyes has drastically decreased and is almost completely unnoticeable. She helped me find ways to resolve my under eye swelling without ever cutting into my face, which I am grateful for. Dr. Gupta is a compassionate doctor that is willing to listen to your concerns and help develop a plan with you to achieve your everlasting facial goals in a natural way."*

For those whose festoons persist and for whom surgery is indicated, I have a detailed discussion of my approach, not just to treat their festoons but to consider simultaneous repair of coexistent changes in the lower lid that may be contributing to festoon formation. Moreover, if there are upper lid and brow changes, then repair of structures below the eyes may make changes above the eyes look worse or unbalanced. I explain in detail my technique and the location of all surgical incision sites. In essence, a comprehensive periorbital rejuvenation plan must be presented to the patient as an option. The patient should feel well informed and not rushed into any decision-making as the psychological preparedness required for a procedure often takes time.

When the patient is ready to schedule the surgery, my office follows a strict protocol to ensure a smooth course for the patient. A written set of preoperative and postoperative instructions (detailed later in this book) are sent to the patient. Out of town patients are advised that they can fly back home as early as two days postoperatively since all sutures are self-dissolving. As all procedures are performed in the office under local anesthesia, there is no need for preoperative lab or blood workup provided that the patient is in stable health and there is no history of a bleeding diathesis. Patients are advised that they will be in no pain during the procedure and most patients sleep through it after the oral sedative has taken effect. Postoperative discomfort is minimal and alleviated with Tylenol® and a low dose of a painkiller if necessary. The next morning, most patients do not experience any pain. Immediately following the procedure, a special flesh-colored dressing is applied around the eyes (no bandages over the eyes), preempting the need for cold compresses or specialized nursing care. Swelling and bruising for most patients is largely resolved by two weeks, after which makeup or concealer may be applied to cover any residual bruising. Limited exercise is permitted after two days and full exercise after one week. Patients are informed that the final result will not be realized for a full year but they will begin to appreciate the early result within a few weeks. My staff and I reassure patients that we are embarking on this year-long journey with them and that we will guide them through every step of the way.

At the time of this writing, my patients have enjoyed being festoon-free for up to 15 years! Alas, successful, long-term management of festoons is possible, but it is predicated on addressing coexistent eyelid changes and a holistic, team approach that includes the festoon surgeon, other specialists, as well as the patient to modify triggers.

Chapter 8
Special Topic:
Festoons from Autologous Fat Grafts

Fat is rich in stem cells and growth factors. When it is harvested from a donor site like the abdomen or thighs and grafted into burned or scarred areas, it can successfully promote wound healing and improved tissue health. When fat is injected into the face for replenishment of lost volume, it serves as a powerful, long-lasting, and natural modality to volumetrically "lift" the face (with or without a surgical facelift) and to rejuvenate the skin.

When fat is injected in or around the delicate skin of the lower eyelid/cheek junction (LCJ) areas, however, there may be untoward consequences. Over the last 15 years, numerous patients have been referred to me who developed festoons after undergoing fat grafting (with or without a facelift) months or years earlier into these zones. I am not suggesting that festoons occur in every recipient of fat grafts in the LCJ or high cheek areas, but my clinical experience is concerning enough to warrant further studies to assess the incidence rate with respect to exact injection location(s), quantity of fat injected, and concurrent facial surgeries such as blepharoplasty or facelift. I propose several mechanisms of festoon formation in such individuals. First, however, it is important to understand how injected fat assimilates into its new milieu. Fat grafts are living tissue harvested from one part of the body and injected into another. In order for this freshly transplanted graft to survive, it must establish a blood supply to receive oxygen and vital nutrients. Otherwise, the fat cells will die or necrose and the body will metabolize and clear them through the circulation, a process called resorption. In fact, every surviving adipocyte or fat cell requires its own capillary bed (see Figure 5), a process called neovascularization, and this robust but helter-skelter network is mediated by an inflammatory (cytokine) cascade.[11-13]

FIGURE 5:
FAT GRAFT STOICHIOMETRY

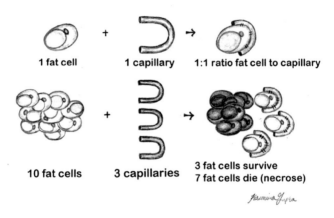

In areas of the face or body where the skin is thicker, the fat/vessel/cytokine complex translates to improved "volume" and skin health. In the LCJ, however, the skin is too thin to mask the increased fluid volume extravasating from the new, leaky, thin-walled blood vessels that course through the fat. This, coupled with the strong, impermeable zygomatic cutaneous ligament (ZCL) that prevents the fluid from traversing down by gravity into the thicker part of the cheek, leads to pooling of the fluid in the most dependent area of the upper face—namely, the prezygomatic space (PZS), with resultant festoon formation. During surgery, I have noted not only hypervascularity within the fat itself but also engorgement of surrounding feeder vessels. Secondly, the greater quantity of fat injected as well as the larger size of the fat grafts (as compared to HA fillers) have the potential to physically impede the delicate lymphatic channels in the lateral face that drain fluid away from the eye and malar regions (see Figure 2). This blockage then results in backup of fluid in the PZS which may also cause or exacerbate festoons.

Lastly, injected fat assumes the personality and characteristics of its home, or donor site. If the patient gains weight in the donor area such as the thighs or abdomen, this will be reflected in expansion of the fat graft in the face and its capillary network as well! Fat graft recipients may note that their faces may swell or shrink with weight gain or weight loss, respectively. With respect to festoons the same may happen.

The management of fat-induced festoons is extremely tedious and challenging. As previously stated, areas where fat is injected are hypervascular and there is significant bleeding despite radiosurgical or laser cauterization. Fat grafts are permanently tethered to the undersurface of the skin and to the surrounding tissues, and there is no reversing agent for their removal. Thus, all injected fat in the cheeks, midface, and under eye areas contributing to the festoons must be removed. Not so easy! As the fat is firmly adherent to the skin, great caution must be exercised to prevent buttonholes in the skin. For fat-induced festoons, I almost always couple festoon repair with a transcutaneous lower blepharoplasty for maximum exposure and access to the injected fat in the lower lid and midface regions. In the hard to access high cheek area, I employ a Nd:YAG (Acculift™ 1444 nm wavelength) laser with a 3 mm laser fiber inserted through the MIDFACE opening to liquefy the injected fat followed by aspiration with a cannula. This laser has the added bonus of tightening the skin from underneath by stimulating collagen production. I have used deoxycholic acid (Kybella®) on a few patients to reduce injected or natural fat in the malar regions, but have discontinued its use after a recent case report showed it may lead to lasting nerve damage.[14]

After thorough removal of all accessible injected fat, the lower lid blepharoplasty with removal of excess skin and herniated orbital fat (if indicated) and eradication of the festoon with my MIDFACE technique are performed.

The patient presentation below demonstrates below how "surprises" are often discovered during surgery despite thorough history-taking.

PATIENT 11:
PHOTOGRAPHS WITH FLASH, INTRAOPERATIVE VIEW

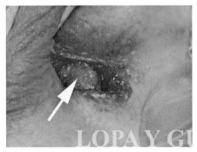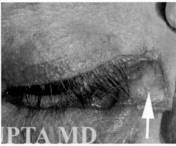

This patient was scheduled for MIDFACE alone (she had already undergone lower lid blepharoplasty elsewhere) to resolve her HA filler festoons. During the procedure, however, injected fat was surprisingly encountered, as depicted by the arrow in the left photograph. To successfully remove all injected fat, a decision was made to perform a lower lid blepharoplasty simultaneously. Fat was noted across the entire lid and tethered to the skin (arrow in right photograph); it took several hours to meticulously tease off the fat to ameliorate her festoons.

PATIENT 11:
PHOTOGRAPHS WITH FLASH, CLOSEUP VIEW

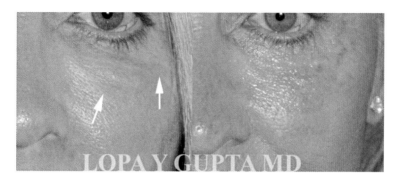

The left photograph demonstrates the extent of the presumed HA filler festoons (arrows). The right photograph is two years after MIDFACE, lower lid blepharoplasty, and removal of injected autologous fat.

Chapter 9
Special Topic:
Festoons from Hyaluronic Acid Fillers

Hyaluronic acid (HA) injections in the tear troughs and cheeks are *the leading cause of festoons in my practice*. Festoons may occur immediately, weeks, months, or even *years* after injection! They may present after serial injections or after even a solitary injection. With the ever-increasing demand for injectable fillers to address volume loss changes as a "quick fix" without surgery, it is imperative for medical professionals to understand how HA fillers work biochemically, to recognize short-term and long-term pitfalls, and to promptly manage their potential complications. Doing so will not only optimize aesthetic outcomes and safety for our patients but also *prevent* unnecessary complications such as festoon formation.

Hyaluronic acid was first isolated from the vitreous humor in the bovine eye by Meyer and Palmer in 1934[15] and its structure was described by Meyer and Weissman in 1953.[16] HA is a complex carbohydrate composed of a chain of two alternating sugar units (D-glucuronic acid and N-acetylglucosamine groups). In fact, a single molecule of HA may contain up to 25,000 repeating sugars! It is very hydrophilic, or water-loving, and can bind up to 1,000 times its weight in water. Scientists have subsequently discovered HA in our skin, joints, muscles, and organs. HA's hydrophilicity and large size enable it to subserve important biologic roles such as hydration, joint lubrication, volumization, and scaffolding for blood vessel formation and fibroblast migration.

FIGURE 6:
HYALURONIC ACID, A SOLITARY UNIT

Hyaluronic acid

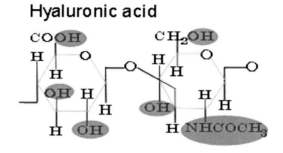

Glucuronic Acid   N-Acetylglucosamine
(Colored areas denote water binding regions)

When it comes to the biologic functions of HA, size matters! Large HA molecules, which are greater than 1,000 kilodalton (kDa) in size *suppress* inflammation and new blood vessel formation. On the contrary, HA polymers smaller than 20 kDa tend to *promote* inflammation and neovascularization.[17,18]

More than 50% of the total body HA is found in the epidermis, dermis, subcutis, and the extracellular matrix of our skin. The amount of HA produced by the body declines with age. This contributes to skin aging and wrinkle formation due to volume loss, dehydration, and decreased elasticity.[19] Natural HA has a half-life of about 24 hours before it is broken down by an enzyme called hyaluronidase. In contrast to collagen, the chemical structure of HA is identical across different species,[20] preempting the need for skin allergy testing prior to injection. Thus, natural HA has unique features that make injected HA an ideal filler for anti-aging purposes. Its hydrophilicity makes it a perfect substance to hydrate and volumize various parts of the face. Its ability to be degraded by an enzyme makes it a reversible filler in situations where too much has been injected or it has been injected into an undesirable location.

Commercially available HA was first extracted from rooster combs by Balazs in 1979.[21] It was called Healon®, or sodium hyaluronate, which was a viscoelastic used during ophthalmic surgery to maintain or replenish intraocular volume. HA is now being produced by bacterial (Streptococcus) fermentation under sterile laboratory conditions. After Restylane® and Juvederm® received FDA approval in 2003 and 2006, respectively, over 120 filler products entered the market; 80% of all fillers are HA-based. There are also non-cosmetic uses for HA, which include topical skin care, osteoarthritis treatment, intraocular surgery, and vesico-ureteral reflux. A recent analysis by Grand View Research valued the global market for HA products at around $9.4 billion in 2022, escalating to $16.8 billion by 2030 with a compound annual growth rate (CAGR) of 7.54%![22]

With the multitude of HA fillers on the market, scientists have studied various attributes of each filler to define its clinical indication, ease of injection, degree of tissue filling, longevity, clinical appearance, and potential side effects. As noted previously, naturally occurring *liquid* HA undergoes rapid degradation. For an HA filler to resist enzymatic breakdown, it must be converted into a *gel* by the process of crosslinking the polymer chains. Thus, the greater the degree of crosslinking, the greater the longevity of the HA product and the longer it can maintain its shape. Researchers also analyze rheological (flow and deformation) properties using the shear test, flow test, and compression test.[23] Shear stress is horizontal or torsional in nature and if the filler can resist deformation, it has a high G prime (G') value, which is a measure of the elastic modulus or stiffness of the gel. Thus, high G' fillers are best for deep volumization but may be harder to inject and more painful. On the contrary, weaker gels with low G' are better suited for thin-skinned or more sensitive areas like tear troughs or lips. The flow test measures the viscosity of the gel. The lower the viscosity, the more readily an HA filler can flow and spread across tissues. Cohesivity, which is the ability of the filler to stay bound together, also plays a role in gel behavior as a low value makes it easier to fragment and move around and mold after injection. The compression test measures the vertical or normal force (F_N) on the gel, which is the force applied by the gel perpendicularly to its surface when it is compressed. F_N allows the gel to resist flattening of the product from pressure caused by skin tissues, allowing the injected area to remain projected during the lifespan of the product. The higher the F_N, the greater the capacity of the filler to project or protrude skin tissues.

Every injector should have a basic understanding of these essential properties of HA fillers to have a working knowledge of which filler to use on any given part of the face to optimize outcome and minimize risk. Nonetheless, it is important for the patient and doctor to be cognizant of potential complications associated with HA fillers. Although rare, vision loss may ensue if filler is inadvertently but forcefully injected into the arteries located between the brows (glabella), tear troughs (under eyes), nasolabial folds, or temples as these arteries anastomose or connect with ophthalmic arteries. The filler travels backwards and obstructs the ophthalmic artery or one of its branches. In a 2015 study by Belezany, of the 98 cases of vision loss reported worldwide, blindness occurred more commonly with autologous fat (47.9%) versus HA filler (23.5%).[24] Other adverse effects of HA filler include necrosis (tissue loss after inadvertent vascular injection), Tyndall effect (bluish discoloration from superficially injected HA that scatters light striking it), infection, reactivation of herpes simplex virus (cold sore), hematoma, and nodules. Most, if not all, of these complications can be avoided or quickly addressed with knowledge of anatomy, knowledge of individual HA filler properties, availability of hyaluronidase (reversing enzyme), and slow, gentle, and careful injection technique.

One of the most dreaded complications of HA filler, festoons, typically occur after sequential or overzealous HA filler injections in the cheek, LCJ, or tear trough area. I have had plenty of patients, however, who manifested festoons after a solitary injection of HA filler years earlier—despite no family history or prior surgical procedures. I make this assertion because I note the presence of the gelatinous filler intraoperatively, as demonstrated by the photographs below:

PATIENT 12:
PHOTOGRAPH WITHOUT FLASH

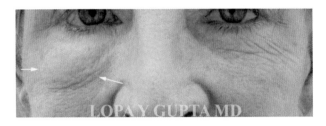

This patient has been suffering from a large HA filler-induced festoon on her right side (arrows) for several years, causing her to go into social isolation. Despite several sessions of reversing enzyme, the festoon has persisted. Note the asymmetry between the two sides with respect to dissolution of the filler.

PATIENT 12:
INTRAOPERATIVE PHOTOGRAPH

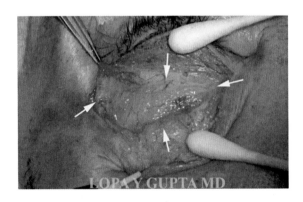

An intraoperative photograph of the patient shown above depicts enzyme-resistant, encapsulated filler that appears shiny and gelatinous (arrows) during open surgery. This trapped filler was causing her large festoon and chronic eyelid edema and was successfully removed with radiosurgery.

Such experiences over the past two decades have taught me that HA fillers do not "go away" after injection. *There is almost always residual filler of varying amounts* in different parts of the face and between the two sides of the face. After serial HA injections, some filler may become encapsulated, rendering it impenetrable to exogenous enzyme administration. An interesting in vivo study conducted in rats by Fernandez-Cossio and Castaño-Oreja in 2006 revealed that subcutaneous injection of Restylane® created an acute inflammatory response within the first four weeks and that by eight months, the implanted filler became "walled off from the surrounding tissue by a capsule consisting of collagen and fibroblasts" with little evidence of biodegradation. Within the implant capsule, there was minimal inflammation or connective tissue formation.[25] To extrapolate this data from the animal model to our faces and validate it by my clinical experience, filler can persist for years beyond injection in one or two ways. First, filler that is walled off or encapsulated becomes impenetrable to natural or injected enzymatic degradation and may become a large hydrophilic unit despite lack of inflammation within the capsule itself. Second, filler that is not walled off is subject to endogenous enzymatic degradation into smaller sugar molecules. These moieties, especially after serial injections, can accumulate and may persist for years, acting as water magnets and mediators of chronic inflammation, new blood vessel formation, and hyperpigmentation with dark circles.

Tarun's Story:

> *"One of the best cosmetic surgeons out there! I have had a long road dealing with hyperpigmented/dark eye circles my whole life; it is due to my race and genetics. I have visited several doctors beforehand, including two dermatologists before her. A third dermatologist recommended that I see her. I wish I knew about her from day one! The first dermatologist put fillers around my eyes, which did not correct the problem and made my hyperpigmentation look worse. He then applied five sessions of a laser that did not work on me. He said there were no other lasers out there that would work on me. I saw a second dermatologist that applied a different laser and did provide some benefits. I made a two hour trip to see Dr. Gupta based on a referral from a third dermatologist. She is well known to the medical community in regards to her ocular work. She has almost fixed me (only three months in and expect to get better over the next several months). She removed the filler, applied threading, injected PRP, and applied her Fraxis laser which has helped tremendously. Second visit, she applied the laser again. I just had my third laser session and feel like it looks about two thirds better from day one and expected to still get better! She is worth the trip and the cost! I probably wasted a few grand beforehand with others. I definitely highly recommend her! She takes the time with you. She and her staff are great, caring, personable and so friendly!"*

Sustained volume increase from HA's hydrophilic effects can be beneficial, especially in parts of the aging face where the skin is thicker (chin, nasolabial folds, marionette lines) or where the edema is localized (lips, temples). The caveat, however, is that the practitioner *must understand and recognize that HA fillers and their effects accumulate over time* and that serial, overzealous injections may lead to distortion of normal facial features.

HA-mediated volume increases in thin-skinned areas like the lower lid and PZS, however, can be unsightly. Just about every patient with an HA filler-induced festoon experiences increased festoon size with low pressure (flying in a plane or skiing), after drinking alcohol or eating a salty meal the night before, or during an upper respiratory infection. This is because low atmospheric pressure, alcohol, salt, and infection potentiate the hydrophilic effects of the retained HA filler residing in the high cheek, malar, and under eye areas—all of which allow gravity-dependent drainage of excess fluid into the ZCL-limited PZS where festoons occur.

Management of HA filler-induced festoons is complex but can be highly successful with excellent long-term results. My treatment algorithm begins with a conservative approach. After a thorough history and physical exam, I perform injections of the enzyme, hyaluronidase, into all contributory areas including the cheeks, midface, and under eyes with an advanced cannula (needle-less) technique to reverse the filler safely and with virtually no bruising. If festoons resolve completely after 2-3 weeks and the skin has retracted (tightened on its own), then no surgery is indicated and the patient is advised to abstain from future HA fillers in that region. If there is a partial response, repeat enzyme injections may be performed. Fillers that are highly cross-linked, or with a high concentration of HA, are harder to dissolve.[26,27] If there is no response to enzyme, the filler has likely become encapsulated. In such cases, other non-surgical options to either tighten the skin envelope or camouflage the festoon include laser resurfacing with Er:YAG or, fractionated CO_2, microneedling with and without radiofrequency, thread-lifting with large bore (18 gauge) dissolvable polydioxanone threads, and deep, supraperiosteal injections of Radiesse® (calcium based filler) to elevate the skin and deeper tissues of the midface and cheek. These remedies are usually short-term, lasting less than a year with varying efficacies. Lastly, if MIDFACE festoon surgery is indicated, it is important to discuss the possible need for adjunctive lower lid blepharoplasty if skin elasticity has been compromised by bouts of edema and stretching from HA filler-induced fluid shifts. During combined surgery, I often note extensive hypervascularity suggestive of chronic inflammation. This is especially noticeable just under the skin flap (see photograph below) and associated with filler dispersed in all directions. The tissues are "boggy" from the chronic fluid influx and the edema extends all the way up along the side of the nose-engorged angular veins and a prominent Tyndall effect. Important components of these procedures include meticulous cauterization of extraneous blood vessels, removal of all HA filler, dehydration of all layers of the festoon sponge, and removal of excess lower lid/festoon skin *without inducing lid retraction.*

Below are representative photographs of a patient who suffered from HA-induced festoons and swelling issues prompting consultation and treatment as per my aforementioned protocol. These photos also highlight the importance of examination and photography from multiple angles.

PATIENT 13:
ALL PHOTOGRAPHS WITH FLASH, CLOSEUP VIEW

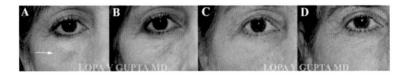

From left to right: (A) Large HA filler festoon (arrow) with elevation and Tyndall effect. (B) Two months after the first hyaluronidase injection with resolution of the mound and Tyndall. (C) Several months later, the festoon recurred near the nose from retained filler (better seen in oblique view). Despite two more enzyme sessions, the festoon persisted as shown, 13 months later. (D) Five months after upper/lower blepharoplasty and MIDFACE.

PATIENT 13:
ALL PHOTOGRAPHS WITH FLASH, OBLIQUE VIEW

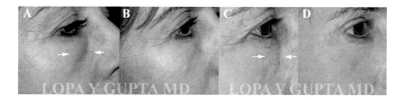

From *From left to right: (A) HA filler festoon with Tyndall (between arrows). (B) Two months after the first enzyme injection with resolution of the festoon and Tyndall. (C) Persistence of nasal festoon despite two sessions of enzyme injections, 13 months later. (D) Five months after upper and lower blepharoplasty and MIDFACE.*

PATIENT 13:
INTRAOPERATIVE VIEW

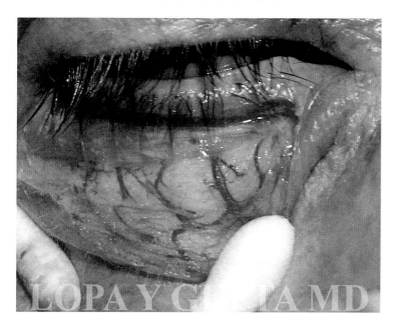

Intraoperative photograph of above patient with engorged vessels under the skin flap. This is a common finding I observe in such patients, demonstrating a robust hypervascularity and chronic inflammatory response triggered by HA filler.

Chapter 10
Special Topic:
Festoons from Chronic Rhinosinusitis (CRS)

I am seeing an increasing number of festoon patients presenting with puffy, fluid-laden upper lids and lower lids. Before considering eyelid or festoon surgery for such patients, it is necessary to rule out nasal or sinus disease as a source of this fluid. To do so, I recruit the expertise of an otolaryngologist (ENT surgeon), *especially in those without a history of HA filler or prior facial surgery.* I have had patients in whom festoons were ameliorated or eradicated with proper nasal or sinus management. Even for patients for whom festoon surgery is undertaken, proper education, evaluation, and management of coexistent nasal or sinus disease is paramount in obtaining an optimal surgical result as well as in minimizing the recurrence rate.

In humans, the eyes are surrounded by four paired paranasal sinuses, which are hollow, air-filled cavities. Other than a thin layer of mucus, the sinuses are empty. The maxillary sinuses are the largest and are situated below the eyes, while the second largest, the frontal sinuses, are located above the eyes. Between the eyes lie the delicate ethmoid sinuses toward the front and the sphenoid sinuses toward the back (Figure 7).

FIGURE 7:
PARANASAL SINUSES

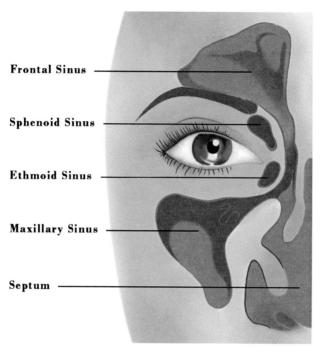

Frontal Sinus

Sphenoid Sinus

Ethmoid Sinus

Maxillary Sinus

Septum

The presumed functions of the sinuses include protecting the eye and brain from external trauma by acting as shock absorbers, lightening the relative weight of the bony skull, and serving as resonant chambers for speech.

The entire respiratory tract, which includes the sinuses, nose, mouth, throat, airways, and lungs, is lined by a mucus membrane that secretes mucus and contains hair-like projections called cilia. Mucus not only protects and lubricates the lining of the respiratory tract, but it also traps bacteria, viruses, toxins, and allergens (dust, pollen) so that the air we breathe is screened and purified before it reaches the lungs. The trapped mucus is then swept away by the cilia into the nose or down the throat where it is swallowed. On occasion, noxious irritants in the respiratory tract stimulate automatic reflexes such as coughing or sneezing to quickly remove unwanted particles from the lungs or nose, respectively.

The mucus from the sinuses drains into the nose through tiny openings called ostia, or meatuses, and aids in regulating the temperature and the humidity of the air we breathe. In addition, each nasal cavity has three scroll-shaped structures called turbinates, which increase the surface area for the air to be adequately heated and moistened. The rich blood supply in the nose also assists with quickly warming the air. The nasal septum divides the nose into two cavities. In each cavity, there are three meatuses through which the sinuses and tear duct (nasolacrimal duct) drain. This is why our nose runs when we cry.

Some anatomic obstacles that lead to decreased air inflow and decreased sinus drainage from compromised meatal openings include deviated nasal septum (the dividing wall of the nose leans to one side with a compromise on that side), turbinate hypertrophy (enlargement of the turbinate tissue fronds), and nasal polyps (small tissue outgrowths in the nasal cavity). Nasal polyps may be present in patients with aspirin sensitivity, cystic fibrosis, asthma, or hay fever after repeated intense histamine-mediated inflammatory attacks to allergens such as pet dander, dust mites, or pollen.

The sinuses are prone to infection and inflammation. Obstruction of the pathway from the sinus to the nose may lead to backup and buildup of mucus in the respective sinus, which, due to its stationary status, or stasis, renders it more susceptible to infection and further inflammation. Thus, a vicious cycle may ensue, wherein the blockage leads to more secretion. This fluid accumulation in the sinus results in a condition called sinusitis. Depending on the etiology of the sinusitis (infectious, inflammatory, allergic), symptoms may range from headache, fever, nasal congestion, facial tenderness over the sinuses, purulent discharge (yellow or green pus), difficulty breathing, sneezing, itching, runny nose, postnasal drip, reduced sense of smell and taste, puffy eyes, to FESTOONS!

The duration of symptoms dictate whether the condition is considered acute rhinosinusitis (ARS) or chronic rhinosinusitis (CRS). ARS is inflammation that generally follows infection by a virus, bacteria, or fungus resulting in more mucus production. CRS usually occurs after a series of infections triggered by allergies, asthma, or nasal polyps, leading to inflammation that persists beyond three months.

Evaluation of the patient begins with examination of the nasal cavity by the ENT surgeon to check for enlarged turbinates or septal deviation. Tapping on the sinuses may elicit sinus discomfort. Endoscopic visualization of the nose and sinuses may be performed with a flexible scope attached to a camera. To rule out bacterial or fungal infection, a mucus specimen is obtained from the sinuses and submitted to the laboratory for culture and antibiotic sensitivities. Computed tomography (CT scan) or magnetic resonance imaging (MRI) enable a detailed evaluation of the nose and sinuses when indicated. Lastly, a skin test for allergies may be necessary to rule out an allergic component to the sinusitis.

The treatment of sinusitis begins with medical and conservative measures to manage infection, inflammation, allergies, and mucus buildup. These include antibiotics, inhaled corticosteroids, decongestants, saline nasal spray, saline irrigation, antihistamines and other allergy medications. If these serve to decrease infection, inflammation, allergies, swelling, or mucus accumulation, then sinus drainage may be improved completely or partially, and the patient will feel better symptomatically.

When these therapies do not suffice, the ENT surgeon may recommend a balloon sinuplasty, an FDA-approved procedure to improve symptomatology and sinus drainage. Balloon sinuplasty is minimally invasive, enabling it to be performed in the office as a walk-in, walk-out procedure. A guide wire is advanced through the nostril and into the tight sinus cavity opening, which is subsequently dilated by inflating a small balloon, allowing the impacted sinus to drain better. Endoscopic sinus surgery may be indicated in some patients to remove polyps or drain the sinuses. A patient with a deviated nasal septum may benefit from septoplasty to improve breathing and sinus drainage. Thus, co-management with an ENT specialist and/or an allergist is vital in the holistic management of the festoon patient that presents with symptoms consistent with ARS or CRS.

Chapter 11
Non-Surgical Methods for Festoon Management

In every cosmetic practice, festoon patients are increasing in number. Non-surgical management of festoons is often undertaken by practitioners with varying degrees of cosmetic training and expertise. As previously noted, the first step is reversing enzyme, or hyaluronidase, injections for HA filler-induced festoons.[26,27] The use of a cannula to facilitate enzyme injections can help minimize bruising and swelling. Also previously mentioned is aggressive laser resurfacing, which is predicated on tightening the skin overlying the festoon by removal of the outer layers of skin to stimulate collagen production.[28] If the practitioner is inexperienced or lacks adequate knowledge of laser physics, devastating complications such as ectropion (lower lid is pulled down or retracted), scarring, hyperpigmentation, hypopigmentation, and infection may ensue. Another method is the use of sclerosing antibiotics such as doxycycline or tetracycline. These agents, when injected into the festoon, serve as noxious irritants that trigger an intense inflammatory response. The goal is to create adequate scar tissue to occupy the potential space, thereby limiting fluid accumulation.[29-31] I have never performed nor offered this treatment because of my biased perspective—over the past decade, dozens of patients have come to my office traumatized by the pain, bruising, and swelling associated with each of the three injections—all for naught as the festoons in these patients did not show any improvement. The studies, nonetheless, report promising short-term and long-term (up to 3.6 years) results.[29-31] Another non-surgical method for festoon improvement is microneedling[32] to tighten the skin envelope by stimulating collagen. In my experience, I have not found this method to be particularly efficacious for festoon improvement. Lastly, camouflage tactics with other fillers in the cheeks to decrease the appearance of the festoon have been employed. Unfortunately, injectors who are not knowledgeable of festoons often use HA filler such as Voluma®, Juvederm®, or Restylane® to mask them short-term; long-term, the HA filler increases festoon size and swelling issues. As mentioned previously, my favorite camouflage filler is Radiesse®, which is not water-loving and when injected deep over the cheekbone, works well to elevate the soft tissue complex of the midface and cheek. This treatment yields a modest but visible reduction in festoon appearance but lasts only about 6-12 months, as demonstrated in the following patient example:

PATIENT 2:
ALL PHOTOGRAPHS WITH FLASH

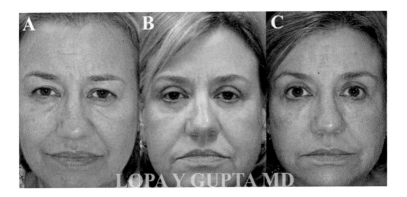

(A) Upper-lower eyelid changes and festoons preoperatively. (B) 6 weeks after laser upper-lower blepharoplasty. Note persistence of festoons as MIDFACE was not yet invented. Deep injections of Radiesse® over her cheekbones were administered to camouflage the festoons, as demonstrated in (C).

PATIENT 2:
ALL PHOTOGRAPHS WITHOUT FLASH

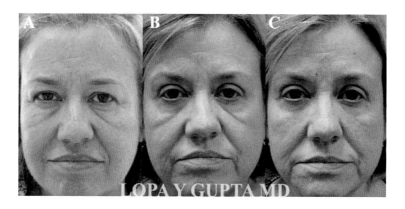

The exact photographs above are shown without flash in this series, facilitating visualization of pre- and post-procedure changes. (A) is preoperative, (B) is six weeks after upper-lower blepharoplasty alone without festoon surgery, showing persistence of festoons, and (C) is immediately after Radiesse® injections.

Unfortunately, there exists no reversing agent for Radiesse®; sodium thiosulfate may show promise as a reversal agent, but no in vivo studies have been published to date. In unskilled hands, however, if Radiesse® is injected too superficially in the tear trough or malar areas, hard, white nodules may develop, as in the case illustrated below.

PATIENT 14:
ALL PHOTOGRAPHS WITH FLASH, FRONTAL VIEW

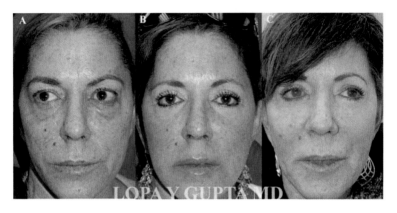

Radiesse® was injected too superficially in the tear troughs by a local doctor in this 57-year-old female, prompting her to go into social isolation for two years. To make matters worse, another doctor injected HA filler over the Radiesse® to camouflage the white deposits. The resultant festoons could not be concealed with makeup, as shown in (A). She underwent successful lower lid blepharoplasty with MIDFACE to address the deposits, lower lid changes, and festoons. In (B), she is nine months postoperative and in (C) her result is maintained five years postoperative.

PATIENT 14:
ALL PHOTOGRAPHS WITH FLASH, CLOSEUP VIEW

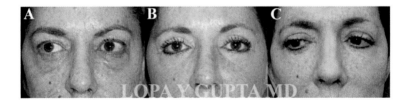

This view enables better visualization of the filler deposits in the tear troughs with an intense inflammatory reaction resulting in chronic redness and swelling in the lower lids. (A) is preoperative, (B) is 9 months postoperative, and (C) is five years postoperative.

PATIENT 14:
ALL PHOTOGRAPHS WITH FLASH, OBLIQUE VIEW

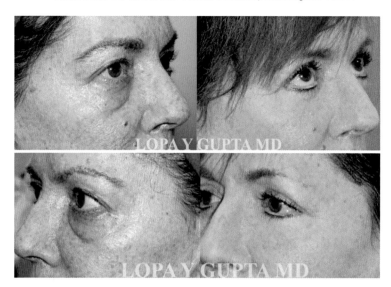

The oblique view depicts nicely the festoons in the preoperative photographs on the left. The result is sustained five years later, as demonstrated in the photographs on the right.

PATIENT 14:
INTRAOPERATIVE PHOTOGRAPHS

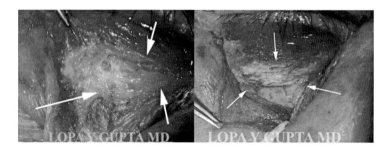

The photograph on the left demonstrates a layer of gelatinous HA filler across the eyelid (arrows). After the HA was destroyed with radiosurgery, a hardened, white layer of Radiesse® was visualized which was also meticulously removed. An intense inflammatory reaction is present, as evidenced by engorged blood vessels in the photographs.

Chapter 12
Surgical Management of Festoons

The surgical management of festoons is very complex and challenging. Most festoon patients are middle-aged or older and often have a complex history of serial fillers or fat injections. Moreover, they often have coexistent lower eyelid changes that *must be taken into consideration* to attain a smooth lower lid cheek junction.[33] Thus, festoons are much more than just swollen cheek mounds and represent only the tip of the iceberg. In a typical patient there exists under the surface a supersaturated fluid "sponge" involving all four layers of the prezygomatic space (PZS) with any or all of the following lower eyelid conditions: edema (swelling), dispersed filler, injected fat tethered to the skin, prolapsed orbital fat (bags), loose skin, loose muscle, thickened muscle, lax ligaments, and prominent tear trough depression. Add to that mixture inflamed, engorged blood vessels from allergies, sinus disease, or leaky neovascularization from filler or fat injections. The festoon specialist must be able to *recognize and surgically treat* each of these potential contributory components for successful long-term management of festoons.

Established methods for festoon repair include direct and indirect approaches. In 1995, Rosenberg[34] described a liposuction technique from a lateral eyelid crease incision to address localized festoons resulting from swollen malar (cheek) fat pads situated just under the skin. This approach may be beneficial in younger patients with hereditary malar mounds, but in the middle aged or older patient, may not serve well as a solitary procedure. It must be coupled with a more comprehensive approach that addresses coexistent lower lid changes or edema in the other layers of the festoon sponge. As previously mentioned, I utilize a modification of this approach with the Acculift™ Nd:YAG 1444 nm laser to liquefy and then aspirate the melted fat from the subcutaneous malar fat pad in select patients. The malar mounds are noticeably reduced but not completely obliterated. The simplest method to eradicate a festoon with multiple components is by direct excision[35], but this method has two potential drawbacks. The long, horizontal incision that is required to completely excise the festoon may lead to an unsightly scar in the center of the face. For younger or darkly complected patients, this may pose an aesthetic issue, especially if the scar is hypertrophic or hyperpigmented. Furthermore, in the absence of a simultaneous lid tightening procedure, there is risk of lower lid retraction given the extent of skin removal.

Thus, subsequent festoon methods steered away from aggressive skin removal and long, direct scars. Instead, they relied on accessing festoons indirectly, such as incisions from the scalp on the side (temporal facelift), from the eyelid above (subciliary and lateral canthal) and from the mouth below (buccal sulcus). From these "less visible" incisions and entry points, a variety of maneuvers could be performed, including aggressive subperiosteal dissections, ligament releases, vertical midface lifting, skin/muscle flaps and soft tissue redraping.[36-39] The goals were to improve the contouring of the lid cheek junction by lifting and resuspending the soft tissues of the midface; to improve the permeability of the previously tight and impervious ligaments to prevent future fluid accumulation, and to tighten and secure the lower lid position to prevent ectropion. Due to the complexity of these procedures, they are usually performed in a hospital or ambulatory surgery center (ASC) operating room under general anesthesia by experienced surgeons with extensive knowledge of eyelid, midface, and facial anatomy. For those who are interested in learning more about these techniques, please refer to the articles cited. Despite such heroics, however, complication rates tend to be high, including damage to the zygomaticofacial nerve, hematoma formation, lower lid retraction, prolonged edema, prolonged recovery times, and, worst of all, high recurrence rates. As Furnas aptly stated in his 1993 article, "Malar mounds have a reputation for persistence despite surgical efforts at correction…"[40]

Chapter 13
M.I.D.F.A.C.E. Explained

Out of necessity for a less aggressive procedure for my burgeoning festoon practice in 2007, I created MIDFACE, an acronym for Mini Incision Direct Festoon Access, Cauterization, and Excision. This moniker is very fitting as the procedure is performed anatomically on the midface. Using advanced laser and radiosurgical methods, MIDFACE is "high tech" but minimally invasive, and is performed *in the office under local anesthesia*. Patients typically walk out of the office minutes after finishing the procedure in little to no pain. The vast majority resume their normal lives within a few weeks. Patient satisfaction rates are very high and the recurrence rate is very low.[4] As the creator of MIDFACE, I am currently the only surgeon knowledgeable and proficient in this procedure but I hope to train other oculoplastic surgeons over the next decade. The aesthetic outcome and long-term success rate of MIDFACE, however, are predicated on multiple prerequisites that took me three decades to learn and master:

1) Advanced knowledge of ocular, eyelid, orbital, nasolacrimal, and midface anatomy
2) In-depth knowledge in the physiology of the optic nerve and vision, lid blink dynamics, dry eye, orbicularis pump, and nasolacrimal apparatus

3) Expertise in lower lid blepharoplasty, especially with simultaneous fat and skin removal with a transcutaneous or subciliary incision approach *without* changing the shape of the eye

4) Expertise in vision-preserving measures in the event of retrobulbar hemorrhage, including canthotomy, cantholysis, pressure lowering drops and medications, anterior chamber paracentesis

5) Expertise in advanced plastic surgery suturing techniques (horizontal mattress, sutures, vertical mattress, buried interrupted, running, running locking, etc) to minimize or preempt scar formation and lower lid retraction

6) Expertise in the use of different types of absorbable and non-absorbable sutures to achieve the desired result for proper external and internal wound healing

7) Expertise in diagnosing and managing a blocked tear duct which could contribute to fluid accumulation in the lower lid/malar areas

8) Expertise in treating dry eyes including placement of punctal plugs, Meibomian gland expression, and intense pulse light (IPL) treatments to improve ocular health prior to and after lower lid surgery

9) Knowledge of all facial injectables in the market (neuromodulators, fillers, fat injections) including their behavior characteristics in each part of the face, longevity, and potential side effects

10) Expertise in injection of facial injectables and their reversing agents in a safe, natural manner in all parts of the face

11) Expertise in cannula methods to safely administer injectables, reversing enzymes to minimize bruising and swelling

12) Expertise in non-surgical management of festoons, including CO_2 and Er:YAG laser resurfacing, administration of reversing enzymes, and supraperiosteal, non-HA fillers (Radiesse®) to "mask" the festoons

13) Expertise in surgical management of iatrogenic (treatment-induced) festoons from fillers (HA, Sculptra®,

silicone), neuromodulators (Botox®, Dysport®, Xeomin®), and injected fat

14) Expertise in surgical management of hereditary festoons resulting from genetics and exacerbated by allergies, sun exposure, pets, age, and gravity

15) Knowledge of aesthetic lasers and radio wave technology including physics, safety, and staff training

16) Appropriate training, certification, and expertise in the safe and successful use of cosmetic lasers and radiosurgery for incisional surgery, fat melting, skin rejuvenation

17) An artistic slant toward surgical and nonsurgical rejuvenation of the face to ensure an aesthetically pleasing and natural result with attention to detail and symmetry

First and foremost, the festoon surgeon must have an in-depth understanding of midface anatomy. The prezygomatic space (PZS) is a complex anatomical area, especially when complicated by lower eyelid changes. The surgeon must be able to distinguish fat that is from the eyelid (herniated orbital fat), versus the subcutaneous area (malar fat pad), versus injected fat (if any), versus the suborbicularis oculi fat pad (SOOF). He/she must know the exact location of the infraorbital nerve centrally and the branches of the facial nerve laterally to prevent numbness in those areas. Prior to performing MIDFACE, I administer hyaluronidase with a cannula to the entire lower lid and festoon complex to reverse as much filler as possible in all HA filler-induced festoons. Although the skin appears looser, there is often a visible, albeit not complete, reduction in eyelid swelling and festoon size with this maneuver alone. The area is then completely numbed with local anesthetic. The 1 cm MIDFACE incision is fashioned precisely in a dynamic orbicularis rhytid in the thin eyelid skin to avoid scarring. After removing an ellipse of skin, the deeper layers of the PZS (SOOF, muscle, subcutaneous fat) are then desiccated and cauterized in the entire festoon complex using high frequency radio waves. This maneuver is performed circumferentially from the small entry point and is continued until there is complete, visible effacement of the festoon. This not only removes the extra fluid from the festoon sponge, but, equally important, it diffusely stimulates collagen production. This minimizes the potential space, tightens the overlying skin and muscle, and possibly strengthens the weak orbicularis retaining ligament. In darker skinned patients, great caution must be exercised in not overheating the skin to prevent post-inflammatory hyperpigmentation (PIH). Deep, absorbable sutures are placed to create an internal wall (collagen) to restrict further, dependent pooling of fluid in the festoon area. The skin sutures are placed meticulously with everted edges to minimize visible scarring. In the postoperative period, I perform light resurfacing treatments with fractionated CO_2 or Er:YAG to enhance skin tone in the lower lid/cheek complex and to minimize incision visibility.

To address coexistent eyelid changes, I perform transcutaneous lower lid blepharoplasty (TCLLB) and MIDFACE simultaneously in one session with radio surgical technology, avoiding scalpel/scissor surgery. The combined procedure begins with a TCLLB and ends with MIDFACE for an optimal result. An incision is made just under the lower lid lash line, and after careful dissection and meticulous hemostasis, prolapsed orbital fat is excised in a conservative fashion to avoid postoperative hollowness. Despite the preoperative enzyme injections, if filler is visualized as a glistening gel, it is destroyed with the heat generated by radio waves. If indicated, unwanted injected fat can be removed with excellent visualization. Loose ligaments can be tightened in older patients, but I generally do not need to perform canthoplasty or canthopexy as my clientele do not wish to alter the shape of their eyes.

This may seem easy and straightforward, but a TCLLB is arguably the MOST technically challenging and risk-laden procedure on the face! Why is this the case? First of all, an eyelid surgeon must always respect and *fear the optic nerve*, which is responsible for vision. Careless surgery may lead to a bleeding vessel, and if this is behind the orbital septum where the fat pads (bags) are excised, a retrobulbar hemorrhage may ensue. If not immediately treated, this can lead to rapid buildup of pressure in the eye and orbit from compartment syndrome, resulting in diminished blood flow to the optic nerve with visual compromise and intense eye pain. A properly trained oculoplastic surgeon can promptly release this pressure by performing a canthotomy and cantholysis to preserve vision. Thus, careful surgery with meticulous attention to hemostasis (no bleeding) is quintessential in *preventing* such a disastrous occurrence. Secondly, an eyelid surgeon is cognizant and always mindful of *preserving* proper eyelid function. The eyelids serve a vital role in covering and protecting our eyes. Normally, we blink 18-20 times per minute to replenish our tear film for clear vision, to keep our eyes moist, and to help pump out environmental toxins from the eyes into the tear ducts and down the nose. During lower lid blepharoplasty, an inexperienced surgeon may remove too much lower eyelid skin, or an aggressive surgeon may perform deep dissections and ligament releases causing the lids to become stiff or partially immobilized by scar tissue. This may result in a condition called ectropion, or lid retraction wherein the lower lid hangs too low and can no longer adequately cover and protect the eye. Since the window remains partially open, the cornea may develop dry spots with a decreased blink rate from lid stiffness. This, in turn, may lead to exposure keratopathy from increased evaporative loss and resultant corneal decompensation. Symptomatically, the patient may experience blurred vision, eye pain, and reflex tearing. It is important to understand that reflex tears are a cry for help as they do not moisturize the eyes! Aside from poor functionality, a droopy lid is unappealing and may lead to poor self-image and depression. If lid retraction persists beyond a few months despite massage, a second, revisional lower lid ectropion repair with or without skin grafting may become necessary to restore form and function. Next, the eyelid surgeon must not violate other important anatomic structures that coexist in the lower lid area, such as the lymphatics in the outer aspect, the inferior oblique muscle in the central aspect, and the lacrimal drainage apparatus (the puncta, canaliculi, lacrimal sac) in the inner aspect of the lower lid. Overly aggressive surgery or insufficient knowledge may result in damage to these vital structures and result in lymphedema (this could make the festoons much worse), double vision, and impaired tear outflow, respectively.

To avoid the devastating complication of lid retraction and an external scar, most eyelid surgeons prefer the transconjunctival route wherein the incision is made inside the eyelid. With this method, however, only fat can be removed and redraped. For patients with advanced skin or tendon laxity, a second, external incision is required for a "skin pinch" removal or lateral canthal tendon plication. Alternately, aggressive laser resurfacing or a chemical peel may be necessary to address skin laxity, with their attendant risks of prolonged redness, swelling, or pigmentary disturbances, especially in darker skin types. Another relative disadvantage of transconjunctival blepharoplasty is the hollowed look from aggressive fat removal, as it is more difficult to gauge the external aesthetic from the internal approach, especially since most surgeons perform such procedures under general anesthesia or intravenous sedation. This precludes intraoperative evaluation of eyelid function (opening and closing) and appearance in the sitting position. Although there is little to no risk of lid malposition and exposure keratopathy (unless aggressive dissections and ligament releases are also performed) from the transconjunctival approach, some patients do experience severe dry eye symptoms likely from direct surgical or edema-induced damage to moisture-producing conjunctival goblet cells or accessory lacrimal glands situated at or near the incision site inside of the lower lid.

A fellowship-trained oculoplastic surgeon, who is also a board-certified ophthalmic microsurgeon, is likely best suited for festoon repair as he/she possesses advanced knowledge and expertise in surgical management of eyelid, lacrimal, and orbital conditions as well as a solid grasp of midface and facial anatomy and techniques. It is very helpful to have a cosmetic slant to the practice as this allows for excellent working knowledge of aesthetic lasers and injectables on the market. Moreover, it is optimal for the festoon patient with lower lid components to have an eyelid surgeon with *extensive experience in transcutaneous blepharoplasty*, who has a negligible rate of lower lid retraction, dry eye complications, hematoma with vision compromise, and incision visibility or scarring. Let's take this a step further. The eyelids are very vascular, and control of bleeding, or hemostasis, is vital to minimize complications. It behooves the patient, therefore, to have a surgeon with expertise in no-scalpel laser or radio wave technology, both of which cauterize blood vessels as they cut through tissues. The increased intraoperative bleeding with scalpel surgery not only increases operative time, but also leads to more scarring, swelling, bruising, pain, and down time postoperatively. Furthermore, scalpel surgery is often performed with electrocautery to control bleeding vessels, which causes significant collateral tissue damage, leading to even more scar tissue. This begs the question: "Why doesn't every eyelid surgeon perform no-scalpel surgery?" One reason is that CO_2 laser or high frequency radio wave surgery entails additional training and costs. As with every new technology, there is a solid learning curve which may take years to master. Most surgeons who trained with scalpel surgery are comfortable with their established method and have very little desire to "relearn" or "unlearn" their technique. To each his own! For those who chose to pursue the non-scalpel path, especially for eyelid surgery, most colleagues would agree that it affords safer, less invasive, and more elegant surgery with less scarring and downtime for the patient.

With optimal hemostasis during laser or radio wave surgery, let's take this a step further. Why would I want to take the patient to the hospital when I can safely perform my procedures in the office? There's no blood work necessary for the healthy patient without a history of bleeding disorder, no extra anesthesia or operating room costs, no waking up with a sore throat with nausea and vomiting from general anesthesia. Thus, for the past 20 years, I have successfully performed all procedures with laser or radio wave surgery in the office under local anesthesia with oral diazepam only. Patients are relaxed, comfortable, and in absolutely no pain throughout. Moreover, I can gauge and fine tune my result on the spot. Under oral sedation, even if the patient is sleeping, the patient can readily follow commands such as looking up, looking down, or sitting up. Having the patient cooperate with these maneuvers helps me achieve a natural result with respect to symmetry, festoon effacement, and appropriate amounts of eyelid skin and fat removal. With a minimally aggressive approach without ligament releases and overzealous skin removal, there is virtually no risk of ectropion and, therefore, a lid plication suture which may permanently alter the shape of the eye (outer corner is pinched or pulled up) becomes unnecessary. Thus, I make every effort to maintain the natural shape of the eyes.

In addition to incisional lasers, the surgeon must also have a solid grasp of the laser physics of the various cosmetic lasers on the market to understand the chromophores (target tissue), laser safety, and the response of each laser to different skin types. While it is helpful to have no-scalpel technology for safer surgery, it is also beneficial to have other adjunctive technological tools at one's disposal to assist intraoperatively, to expedite the post-surgical healing or to enhance the result. For example, the Nd:YAG 1444 nm laser (Acculift™) is essential in melting injected fat; the Er:YAG in decreasing incisional line visibility and scarring; fractional CO_2 in further skin tightening and collagen building postoperatively; and the intense pulse light (IPL) in rapidly decreasing bruising and improving dry eye.

It is also extremely important for the surgeon to possess in-depth knowledge of all injectable agents on the market as festoons are a frequent consequence of many of these. This knowledge is most readily acquired if the surgeon has a sizable injectable practice to really understand the behavior and nuances of each of the agents. Patients often forget about where on their face and when they had certain injections, especially if they were more than a couple years ago, despite thorough history-taking by the surgeon. I have often come across "surprises" during surgery such as Sculptra, silicone, or Radiesse® in addition to the usual HA filler or injected fat. The surgeon must be able to not only visually recognize these substances but also be equipped to remove or reverse them intraoperatively as they may be a source of festoon fluid. Failure to do so may result in a suboptimal result or recurrent festoons.

Going a step further, the surgeon must be an artist as well. As I always tell my patients: "One can rush a surgeon but not an artist!" An artist, by nature, is a perfectionist. This means paying meticulous attention to detail, whether it is in the way the patient is positioned to the way I am holding the laser in my hand to having perfect lighting to making every throw of every stitch "perfect." Moreover, an artistic eye enables the surgeon to visualize the result before surgery. This is critical, because I feel I am always guided by this end result with every step of the procedure.

In summary, a qualified festoon surgeon requires a "perfect storm": specialized training, exquisite knowledge of eyelid and facial anatomy, experience with surgical and non-surgical eyelid procedures and injectables, a well-equipped office with availability of and expertise in radio wave and laser technologies, and an artistic bent are all prerequisites for consistent, safe, and successful outcomes when it comes to management of festoons.

Samille's Story:

> *"I have been going to Dr. Gupta for 7+ years now and have never been disappointed once, despite the huge variety of work I have had done by her (facial reconstructive surgery i.e. festoons, laser hair removal, hair regrowth treatment, Juvederm, etc.). She is honest about her abilities and about how long the process will take, how long the healing will take, and so on. I trust her with my body completely. Of course, every human takes different amounts of time to heal given the varying sensitivities of our face and skin, our age, exposure to sun, and other conditions that have the potential to alter our healing processes. However, Dr. Gupta has a very large understanding of different body types and will be genuine with you about what she thinks is best given your conditions. She is caring, kind, and dedicated to her patients, wanting the absolute best for them. Her staff is great too. They have my utmost trust and confidence."*

Lisa's Story:

"Dr. Lopa Gupta is emphatically the best! Not only in education and medical training from the top schools, but her area of expertise goes beyond a typical surgeon. She specializes in eye surgery and the face. She is not only the best because of her experience, but also her artistic eye, approach, and technique. From the moment you walk in the office it does not feel like just a medical experience, but the highest level of personal, discrete, professionalism, attention to detail, and patience and support to educate you through the process, every step of the way. Often when we are doing research to find the right doctor and the right fit we need a support staff that not only explains things, but goes over it as many times as you need to completely understand the process. Dr. Lopa Gupta is the hidden gem and renowned globally. I know celebrities and top professionals that have sought her services over the years and have all been beyond pleased with the outcome, which is why I entrusted my face to her. Of course, safety precautions, the latest technology in education, and process were all part of my decision. When you ask questions you get answers, when you ask better questions you get better answers, and Dr. Lopa Gupta's medical team raises the standard of what all procedures should be. After I had the face procedure. I not only look refreshed, more rejuvenated, and healthy, but it is beyond my expectation. The procedure is seamless, smooth, and at the highest level of professional practices. When you are entrusting your medical well-being and the outcome of eye surgery or face surgery, you must completely turn it over to the process. My experience was the best. I wish every woman or man that is considering a procedure to have the opportunity to work with Dr. Gupta and her beautiful team. The kindness, warmth, and wisdom of Dr. Gupta and her team are unsurpassed and so appreciated. The process and procedure was once and now I get to enjoy the difference for the rest of my life! I can only say two words, over and over again: thank you Dr. Lopa Gupta, Ann, Angelina and Inelda!"

Chapter 14
Preoperative And Postoperative Instructions

I cannot overemphasize the importance of adhering to both preoperative and postoperative care regimens. In my office, I give each patient a written set of such instructions. The basic idea is that before surgery, the body must be "prepped" to minimize bruising and swelling. This is best accomplished by thickening the blood to allow it to clot quickly and sufficiently. Every individual heals differently, and even the two sides of the same individual can heal differently! Many factors influence how we heal, and to name just a few, they include diet, exercise, sun exposure, medications, vitamins, hereditary bleeding disorders (Von Willebrand's disease, thrombocytopenia, thalassemia, sickle cell, hemophilia), chronic illness (cancer, organ failure), and prior surgery with possible scar tissue or damaged lymphatics. That said, our bodies have a unique, natural rheostat for internal healing and there is really no way to rush the microscopic healing which goes on for about a year. What we *can* modify is the acute phase of clinical healing—that which is apparent to the naked eye in the early postoperative period. The onus is on the patient to comply with the recommended preoperative and postoperative regimen to minimize bruising and swelling as well as to prevent infection, bleeding, scarring, or wound dehiscence. It is also important for the patient to understand that eyelid changes and festoon formation likely happened over *years* and the final result simply cannot be realized in *days*! Patience is a virtue and de-stressing about the healing period may, paradoxically, expedite it.

Before Surgery Instructions:

- Discontinue these medications/supplements 1-2 weeks prior to the procedure to limit bruising:
  - o aspirin, baby aspirin, ibuprofen (Motrin®, Advil®, Aleve®), ginseng, fish oil (omega-3 fatty acids), garlic, ginger, gingko, all vitamin supplements, evening primrose oil, St. John's wort

- Discontinue or limit 1-2 weeks prior:
  - o Salty food, garlic, alcohol, fish, smoking

- Begin these to *decrease* bruising/swelling
  - o Arnica Montana pellets or pills
  - o Bromelain pills or pineapple (natural source of bromelain)
  - o Spinach, kale, collard greens (natural source of Vitamin K)

- Hair treatments must be done prior to the procedure

Day of Surgery Instructions:

- The face should be cleaned and free of makeup, contacts, and eyelash extensions

- Eat a light meal before heading to the office for the procedure

- Wear a loose, button-down shirt to avoid eye/face contact when removing

- A topical numbing cream, an oral sedative, and local anesthetic will be administered for optimal relaxation and no pain during the procedure

- Arrange for a ride to and from the office

After Surgery Instructions:

- Restrict salt and alcohol intake for 1-2 weeks

- Control allergies with antihistamines or nasal sprays

- Optimize sun protection with sunscreen, sunglasses, or hat

- Abstain from makeup for 2-4 weeks. After that time, the operated area should be handled with care without excessive rubbing when applying or removing makeup

- Wear hypoallergenic makeup for the first few months

- Avoid rubbing the operated areas after pet handling. Hands must be washed frequently

- Abstain from future hyaluronic acid or fat injections in the eye/upper cheek areas as festoons will recur

- Use a science-based maintenance eye cream that contains appropriate concentrations of retinol, hyaluronic acid, vitamin C, and other antioxidants

- Abstain from aggressive laser resurfacing, microneedling, or chemical peel treatments in the lid/cheek area for 6 months as they may cause excessive swelling

Recommendations and Future Directions

I would like to offer some words of wisdom to those who have read this book. Always put "ME FIRST" when considering facial rejuvenation:

M: Mental Health
Is this hangup affecting my mental health and everyday life?

E: Expectations
What do I expect to see improved on my face, in order of priority, so that I look natural and refreshed: less puffiness, less hollowness, less darkness, fewer wrinkles, etc.?

F: Finances
What do I want to budget for these facial improvements?

I: Instant Gratification
I would like to see some immediate improvement to make me feel better about what I see in the mirror and what I spend, but I EXPECT my face to be a work in progress. I do not want to do too much too quickly.

R: Risks
Am I aware of the risks involved in facial rejuvenation? I know the doctor will review these with me, but have I done my due diligence?

S: Safety
This is my face, these are my eyes, and I want to feel safe when I have something done. I owe it to myself to invest in a professional who is experienced, knowledgeable, and conservative to give me a result that is natural, safe, and refreshed.

T: Time
How much down time do I have to undergo facial treatments? None? A few days? A few weeks?

After this self-analysis and introspection, here are some salient questions to ask your doctor. If your doctor cannot answer them to your satisfaction, you may want to consult another specialist to feel confident that he/she will be able to help you in the event festoon formation occurs:

Ask Your Doctor:

- Is my condition going to improve with one session or do I need multiple?

- Is the filler likely to stay put in the location where it was injected, or can it be displaced with manipulation (wiping off makeup, washing/drying your face, etc.) or exercise?

- How much swelling/bruising can I expect after, and what are the short- and long-term complications?

- Will my body dissolve the filler completely or in part, and if my body does not dissolve all of the filler, will there be asymmetry between the two sides? Will the residual filler that stays cause issues long- or short-term?

- Have any of your patients had swelling issues after the filler injections, short- or long-term?

- Are you aware of what festoons are, and are you aware that HA fillers in the tear troughs or cheeks can cause festoons in the short- and long-term? If I get festoons from the filler, do you know how to get rid of them?

- What will happen to my skin once the filler is removed? Will the skin tighten up on its own, or will I need surgery?

It is my ardent desire that with increased festoon awareness and knowledge on the part of the patient and doctor, a greater concerted effort will be made to properly manage festoons and ideally, to prevent festoons. As much as cosmetic specialists want to capitalize on patients wanting to look great and as much as patients are willing to spend thousands of dollars on their faces, we must ALL remember that our top priority is to practice "good medicine." Patients and doctors, hopefully, will know better than to do serial HA filler injections around the eye/cheek area and to think twice before fat grafts are placed in these areas. As technology continues to evolve there may be more treatment options and other novel techniques for festoon sufferers, even less invasive than the MIDFACE procedure. Aesthetic rejuvenation, both surgical and non-surgical, is my passion but nothing would give me greater satisfaction than the eradication of iatrogenic festoons.

REFERENCES

1. Khatri KA, Ross V, Grevelink JM, Magro CM, Anerson RR: Comparison of Erbium:YAG and Carbon Dioxide Lasers in Resurfacing of Facial Rhytides. *Arch Dermatol* 1999; 135:391-7.

2. Attachment 15, 510(k) Summary Statement for K963339 the Coherent ULTRAPULSE Carbon Dioxide Surgical Lasers. Page amended November 27, 1996. FDA approval stamped January 22, 1997.

3. The 2007 Plastic Surgery Report, released by the American Society of Plastic Surgeons (ASPS). www.plasticsurgery.org/documents/News/Statistics/2007/pla stic-surgery-statistics-full-report-2007.pdf.

4. Gupta LY, Gupta SG, Bamberger JN, Gupta KR: A Novel, Minimally Invasive Festoon Surgery: Mini Incision Direct Festoon Access, Cauterization, and Excision (MIDFACE): a 12 Year Analysis. *Plast Reconstr Surg* Advance online article DOI: 10.1097/PRS.0000000000010365.

5. Furnas DW: Festoons of orbicularis muscle as a cause of baggy eyelids. *Plast Reconstr Surg* 1978; 61(4):540-546.

6. Kikkawa DO, Lemke BN, Dortzbach RK: Relations of the Superficial Musculoaponeurotic System to the Orbit and Characterization of the Orbitomalar Ligament. *Ophthal Plast Reconstr Surg* 1995; 12(2):77-88.

7. Pessa JE, Garza JR: The malar septum: the anatomic basis of malar mounds and malar edema. *Aesthet Surg J* 1997; 17:11-17.

8. Mendelson BC, Muzaffar AR, Adams WP: Surgical Anatomy of the Midcheek and Malar Mounds. *Plast Reconstr Surg* 2002; 110(3):885-896; discussion 897-911.

9. Muzaffar AR, Mendelson BC, Adams WP: Surgical Anatomy of the Ligamentous Attachments of the Lower Lid and Lateral Canthus. *Plast Reconstr Surg* 2002; 110(3):873-884.

10. Goldman MP: Festoon formation after infraorbital botulinum A toxin: a case report. *Derm Surg* 2003; 29(5): 560-1.

11. Khouri RK Jr, Khouri RK: Current Clinical Applications of Fat Grafting. *Plast Reconstr Surg* 2017; 140(3):466-486.

12. Bucky LP, Percec I: The science of autologous fat grafting: views on current and future approaches to neo-adipogenesis. *Aesthet Surg J* 2008; 28(3):313-321.

13. Evans BGA, Gronet EM, Saint-Cyr MH: How Fat Grafting Works. *Plast Reconstr Surg Glob Open* 2020; 8:e2705. Published online July 14 2020.

14. Pathoulas JT, Demer AM, Kingsley-Loso JL, Farah RS: Lasting marginal mandibular nerve injury following submental deoxycholic acid treatment. *International Journal of Women's Dermatology* 2020; 6(3):232.

15. Meyer K, Palmer J: The polysaccharide of the vitreous humor. *J. Biol Chem* 1934; 107:629-634.

16. Weissmann B, Meyer K: The structure of hyaluronic acid and of hyaluronic acid from umbilical cord. *J Am Chem Soc* 1954; 76:1753-1757.

17. Allison DD, Grande-Allen KJ: Hyaluronan: a powerful tissue engineering tool. *Tissue Eng* 2006; 12:2131-2140.

18. Jagannath S, Ramachandran KB: Influence of competing metabolic processes on the molecular weight of hyaluronic acid synthesized by *Streptococcus zooepidemicus*. *Biochem Eng J* 2010; 48(2):148-158.

19. Ghersetich I, Lotti T, Campanile G, Grappone C, Dini G: Hyaluronic acid in cutaneous intrinsic aging. *Int J Dermatol* 1994; 33(2):119-122.

20. Richter AW, Ryde EM, Zetterstrom EO: Non-Immunogenicity of a Purified Sodium Hyaluronate Preparation in Man. *Int Arch Allergy Appl Immunol* 1979; 59:45-8.

21. Balazs E: Ultrapure hyaluronic acid and the use thereof. US Patent 4 141 973. Issued October 17, 1979.

22. Grand View Research, 2022: Hyaluronic Acid Market Size, Share & Trends Analysis Report by Application (Dermal Fillers, Osteoarthritis, Ophthalmic, Vesicoureteral Reflux), By Region (MEA, EU, North America, APAC), and Segment Forecasts, 2023-2030 Report ID: 978-1-68038-333-1, Grand View Research Inc, San Francisco, USA.

23. Stocks D, Sundaram H, Michaels J, Durrani MJ, Wortzman MS, Nelson DB: Rheological evaluation of the physical properties of hyaluronic acid dermal fillers. *J Drugs Dermatol* 2011; 10(9):974-980.

24. Belezany K, Carruthers JDA, Humphrey S, Jones DJ: Avoiding and treating blindness from fillers: a review of the world literature. *Dermatol Surg* 2015; 41:1097-1117.

25. Fernandez-Cossio S, Castano-Oreja MT: Biocompatibility of two novel dermal fillers: histological evaluation of implants of a hyaluronic acid filler and a polyacrylamide filler. *Plast Reconstr Surg* 2006 117: 1789-1796.

26. Rao V, Chi S, Woodward J: Reversing facial fillers: interactions between hyaluronidase and commercially available hyaluronic-acid based fillers. *J Drugs Dermatol* 2014; 13:1053-6.

27. Jones D, Tezel A, Borrell M: In vitro resistance to degradation of hyaluronic acid dermal fillers by ovine testicular hyaluronidase. *Dermatol Surg* 2010; 36:804-9.

28. Scheiner AJ, Baker SS, Massry GG: Laser management of festoons. In: Masters Techniques in Blepharoplasty and Periorbital Rejuvenation. New York: Springer; 2011: 211-221.

29. Perry JD, Mehta VJ, Costin BR: Intralesional tetracycline injection for treatment of lower eyelid festoons: a preliminary report. *Ophthal Plast Reconstr Surg* 2015; 31(1):50-2.

30. Godfrey KJ, Kally P, Dunbar KE, Campbell AA, Callahan AB, Lo C, Freund R, Lisman RD: Doxycycline injection for sclerotherapy of lower eyelid festoons and malar edema: preliminary results. *Ophthal Plast Reconstr Surg* 2019 35(5):474-7.

31. Chon BH, Hwang CJ, Perry JD: Long Term Experience with Tetracycline Injections for Festoons. *Plast Reconstr Surg* 2020; 146(6):737e-743e.

32. Geronemus RG: Successful Noninvasive Treatment of Festoons. *Plast Reconstr Surg* 2018; 141(6); 977e-978e.

33. Goldberg RA, McCann JD, Fiaschetti D, Ben Simon GJ: What causes eyelid bags? Analysis of 114 consecutive patients. *Plast Reconstr Surg* 2005; 115:1395-1402.

34. Rosenberg GJ: Correction of Saddlebag Deformity of Lower Eyelids by Superficial Suction Lipectomy. *Plast Reconstr Surg* 1995; 96(5): 1061-1065.

35. Einan-Lifshitz A, Hartstein ME: Treatment of festoons by direct excision. *Orbit* 2012; 31(5):303-306.

36. Krakauer M, Aakalu VK, Putterman AM: Treatment of malar festoon using modified subperiosteal midface lift. *Ophthal Plast Reconstr Surg* 2012; 28(6):459-62.

37. Schiller JD. Lysis of the orbicularis retaining ligament and orbicularis oculi insertion; a powerful modality for lower eyelid and cheek rejuvenation. *Plast Reconstr Surg* 2012; 129(4):692-700.

38. Hoenig JF, Knutti D, de la Fuente A: Vertical subperiosteal midface lift for treatment of malar festoons. *Aesth Plast Surg* 2011; 35:522-529.

39. Hamra ST: Building the Composite Face Lift: A Personal Odyssey. *Plast Reconstr Surg* 2016; 138(1):85-95.

40. Furnas, DW: Festoons, mounds, and bags of the eyelids and cheek. *Clin Plast Surg* 1993; 20:367-385.

About The Author

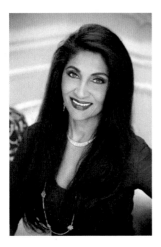

Dr. Lopa Gupta is a Stanford-trained, Board-certified oculoplastic surgeon who, over the past 25 years, has crafted a niche, bespoke practice in no-scalpel eyelid and festoon surgery using laser and radio wave technology. She is the creator of MIDFACE, a minimally invasive procedure that draws festoon sufferers from around the globe to reclaim their faces and lives. MIDFACE is published in the journal *Plastic and Reconstructive Surgery* and has been presented at international conferences.

In 1991, Dr. Gupta married fellow Northwestern Honors Program alum Dr. Mantu Gupta, who is Chair of Urology at Mount Sinai West in New York and one of the leading minimally invasive kidney stone surgeons in the world. They have raised 3 beautiful children, Sarina, Dilan, and Kasmira—their names serving as the inspiration for SaDilKa, a non-profit the family founded 20 years ago for humanitarian missions in impoverished areas.

Dr. Gupta also has a penchant for reading the classics, world travel, interior design, architecture, fashion, singing, dancing, tennis, and doting on her family.

Lopa Y. Gupta, M.D.
Castle Connolly Top Doctor
Board-Certified Oculofacial Plastic Surgeon
Festoon & Laser Eyelid Surgery

Made in the USA
Las Vegas, NV
03 January 2025

66fcff4b-3f6b-4085-a769-35e487ad2d4dR01